HI-TECH HEALTH CARE

3D PRINTING IN HEALTH CARE

by Marne Ventura

BrightPoint Press

San Diego, CA

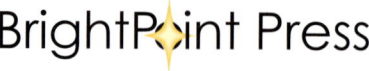

© 2022 BrightPoint Press
an imprint of ReferencePoint Press, Inc.
Printed in the United States

For more information, contact:
BrightPoint Press
PO Box 27779
San Diego, CA 92198
www.BrightPointPress.com

ALL RIGHTS RESERVED.

No part of this work covered by the copyright hereon may be reproduced or used in any form or by any means—graphic, electronic, or mechanical, including photocopying, recording, taping, web distribution, or information storage retrieval systems—without the written permission of the publisher.

LIBRARY OF CONGRESS CATALOGING-IN-PUBLICATION DATA

Names: Ventura, Marne, author.
Title: 3D printing in health care / by Marne Ventura.
Description: San Diego, CA : BrightPoint Press, [2022] | Series: Hi-tech health care | Includes bibliographical references and index. | Audience: Grades 7-9
Identifiers: LCCN 2021009964 (print) | LCCN 2021009965 (eBook) | ISBN 9781678201906 (hardcover) | ISBN 9781678201913 (eBook)
Subjects: LCSH: Medical technology--Juvenile literature. | Medical care--Technological innovations--Juvenile literature. | Three-dimensional printing--Juvenile literature.
Classification: LCC R855.3 .V46 2022 (print) | LCC R855.3 (eBook) | DDC 610.285--dc23
LC record available at https://lccn.loc.gov/2021009964
LC eBook record available at https://lccn.loc.gov/2021009965

CONTENTS

AT A GLANCE   4

INTRODUCTION   6
    SAVING JAMAR

CHAPTER ONE   14
    WHAT IS THE HISTORY OF 3D PRINTING IN HEALTH CARE?

CHAPTER TWO   28
    HOW DOES 3D PRINTING IN HEALTH CARE WORK?

CHAPTER THREE   40
    HOW ARE DOCTORS USING 3D PRINTING TODAY?

CHAPTER FOUR   60
    WHAT'S NEXT FOR 3D PRINTING IN HEALTH CARE?

Glossary   74
Source Notes   75
For Further Research   76
Index   78
Image Credits   79
About the Author   80

AT A GLANCE

- 3D printing was invented in 1983 by American inventor Charles Hull. Today consumers can buy cheap 3D printers for home use. Professional 3D printers used by engineers, scientists, and doctors are more precise and use more types of materials.

- A regular printer creates a single layer of printed matter. 3D printers make objects with many layers.

- Health care experts began using 3D printers in 1999. Instead of ink, these printers use biomaterials.

- Doctors print body parts to repair or replace damaged parts in patients. They implant these parts into patients using surgery.

- Experts have printed and implanted bladder tissue, tracheas, skin, cartilage, and other tissues.

- Orthopedists print artificial joints and implant them in patients. A patient's bones grow into the joint.

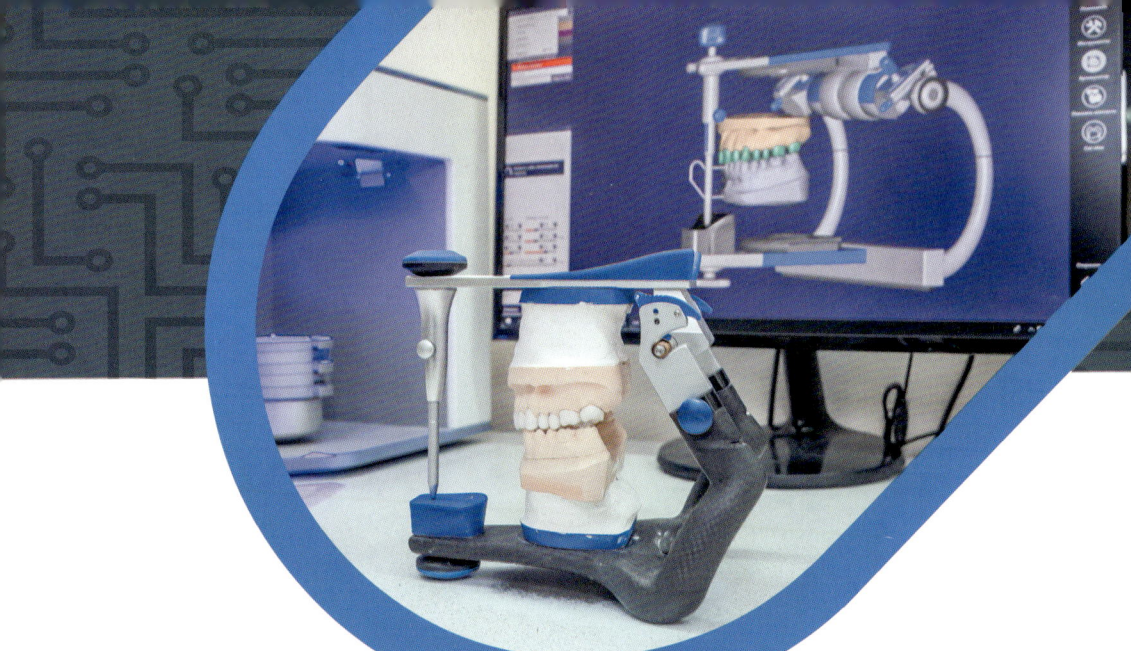

- Experts who make artificial limbs use 3D printing to create body parts that fit their patients just right. These parts are comfortable for patients and are inexpensive to make.

- Medical students and surgeons use 3D printed body parts to practice surgery. Drugmakers test their drugs on 3D printed tissue.

- Scientists hope to make working organs, such as hearts and livers, in the future. This is a challenge because these organs are very complex.

- Working 3D printed organs would benefit patients who need organ transplants.

INTRODUCTION

SAVING JAMAR

Three-month-old Jamar was born with a rare disease. His airway had not developed. It kept collapsing. Doctors attached him to a ventilator. This device pushed air in and out of his lungs. Without it, he might die.

The medical team could repair Jamar's airway with surgery. But it was risky. A machine called a 3D printer might help.

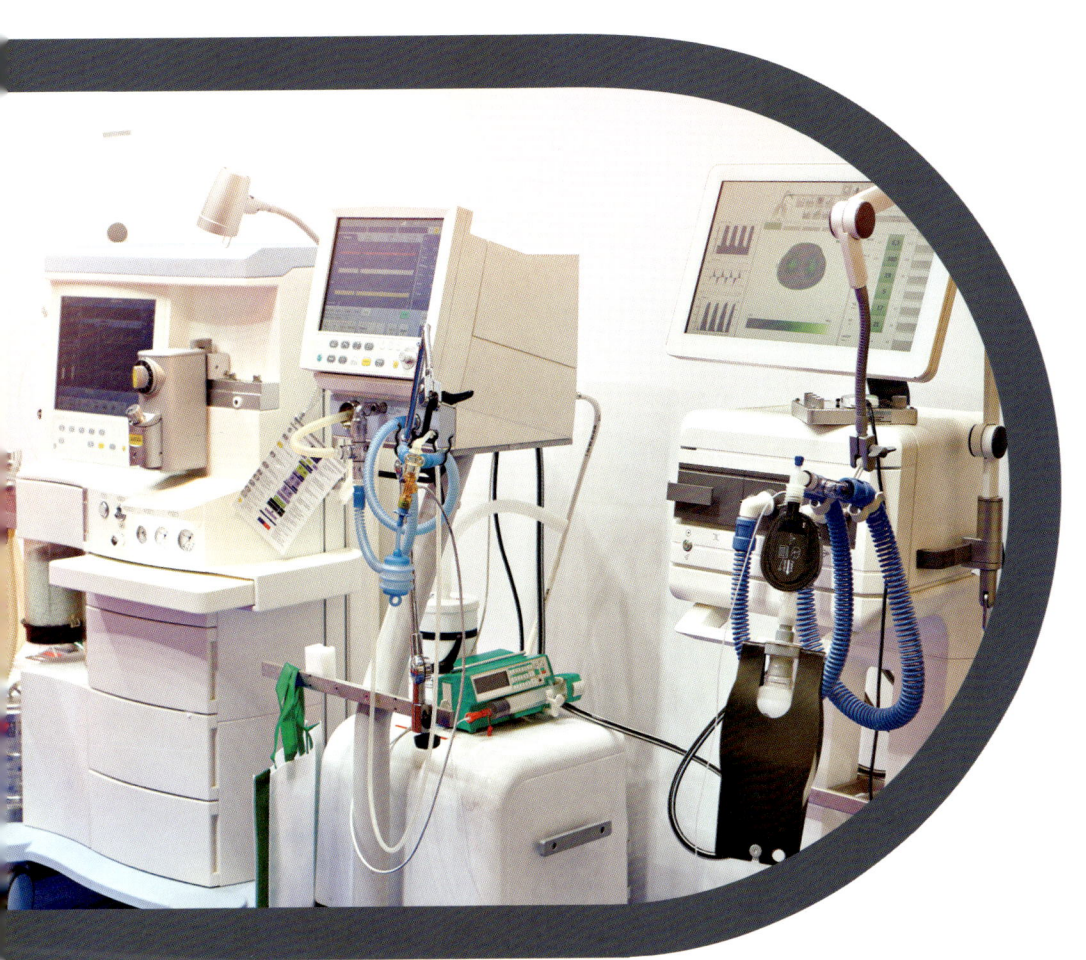

Ventilators help people who have trouble breathing. 3D printed airways can offer a better long-term solution.

The team took X-rays of Jamar's airway.

They used the images to create a design in the same shape on a computer. They sent this design to a 3D printer. The team used suture material as the printing substance. This material is normally used for stitching up wounds. They printed a strong, flexible tube. It was just the right size for Jamar.

The doctors operated on Jamar. They fit the tube around Jamar's weak airway. Now Jamar could breathe without a ventilator. By the time Jamar was three, his airway had developed so that he could breathe on his own. The 3D printed tube gradually dissolved.

A BREAKTHROUGH FOR HEALTH CARE

Jamar is a fictional character. But what happened to him is based in fact. Today,

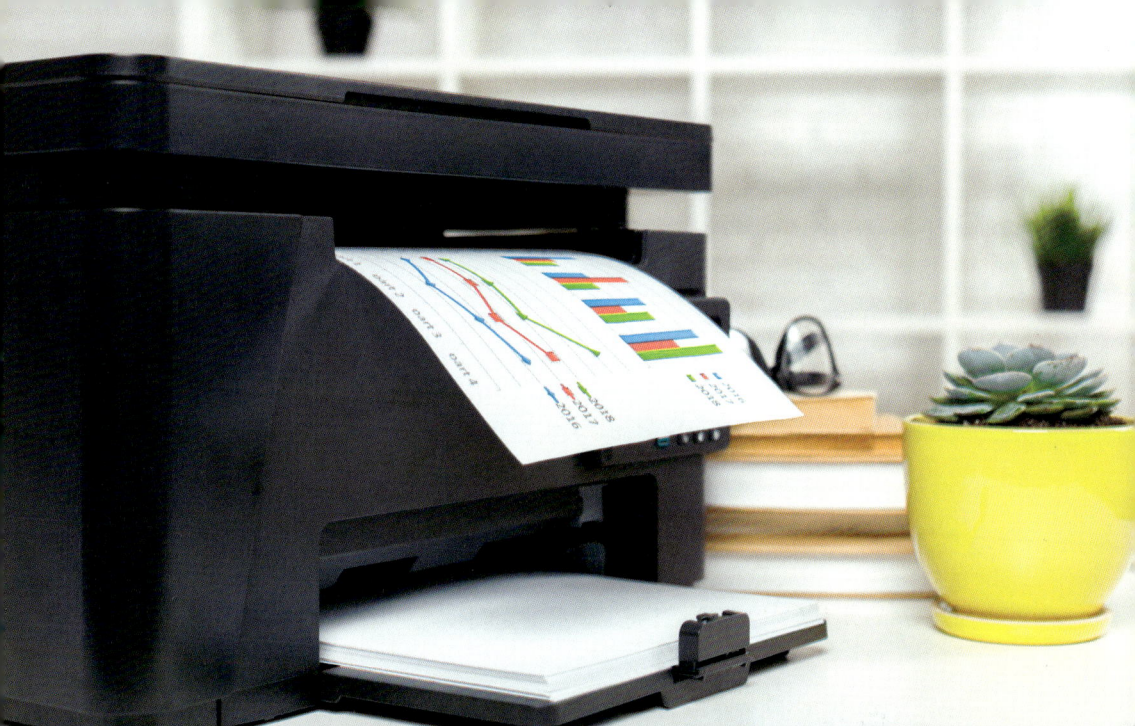

Normal printers produce two-dimensional images on paper.

3D printers in health care are changing people's lives for the better.

Ordinary printers work in two dimensions. A computer sends a file containing words or pictures to the printer. Motors pull a sheet of paper through the printer. Separate motors move a part called the print head from side to side across the paper. Ink sprays in tiny drops from the print head. It lands on the paper and forms the words or pictures. The printed material has height and width. It is flat.

3D printing is similar to printing on paper. But it adds layer after layer to make an object with height, width, and depth. Instead of ink, it uses plastic, metal, or a variety of other materials. After each layer, the printer lowers the object. Then it prints the next layer on top of the last.

Inventors and engineers started printing plastic objects in the 1980s. They improved

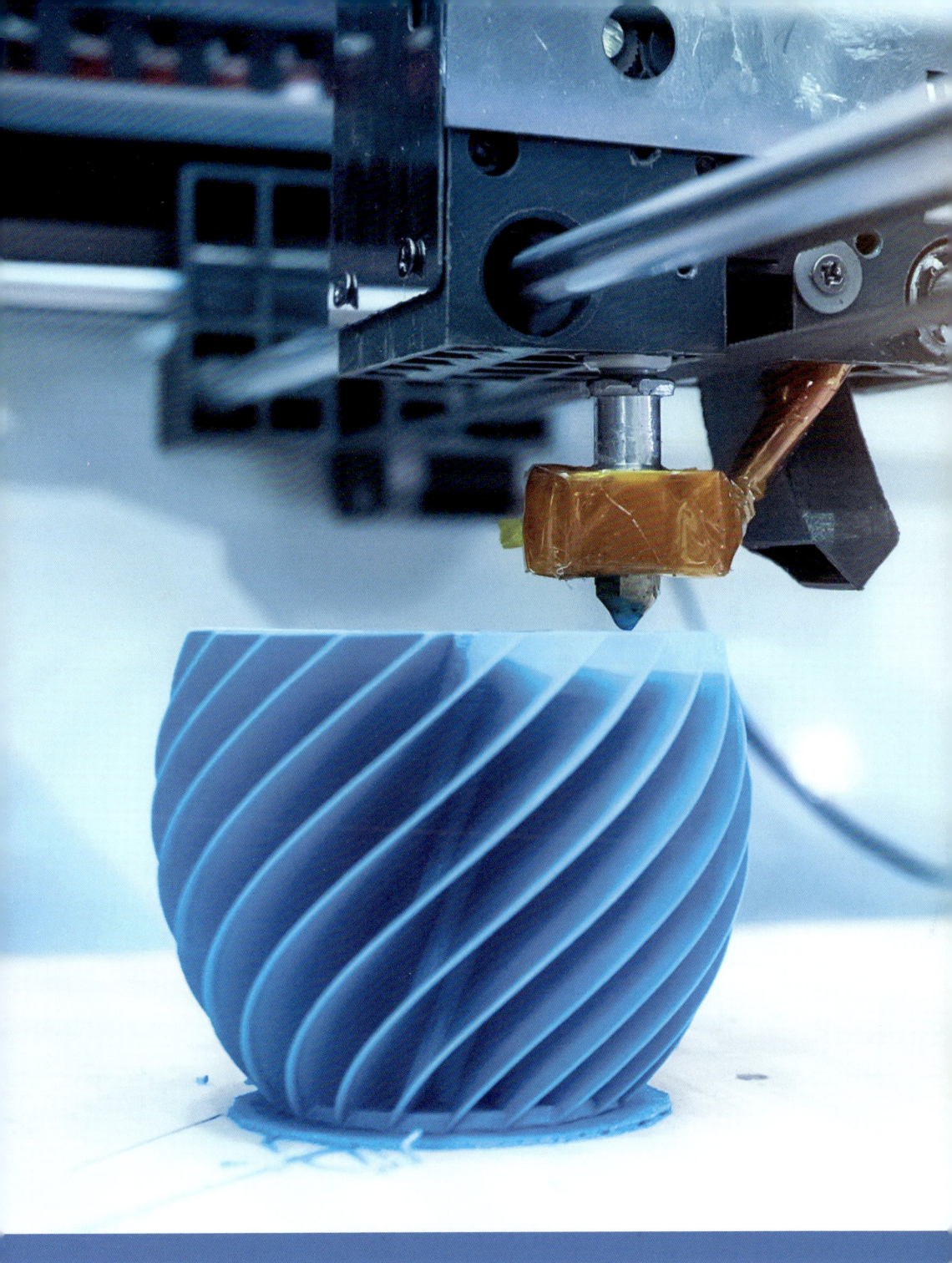

3D printers build objects layer by layer.

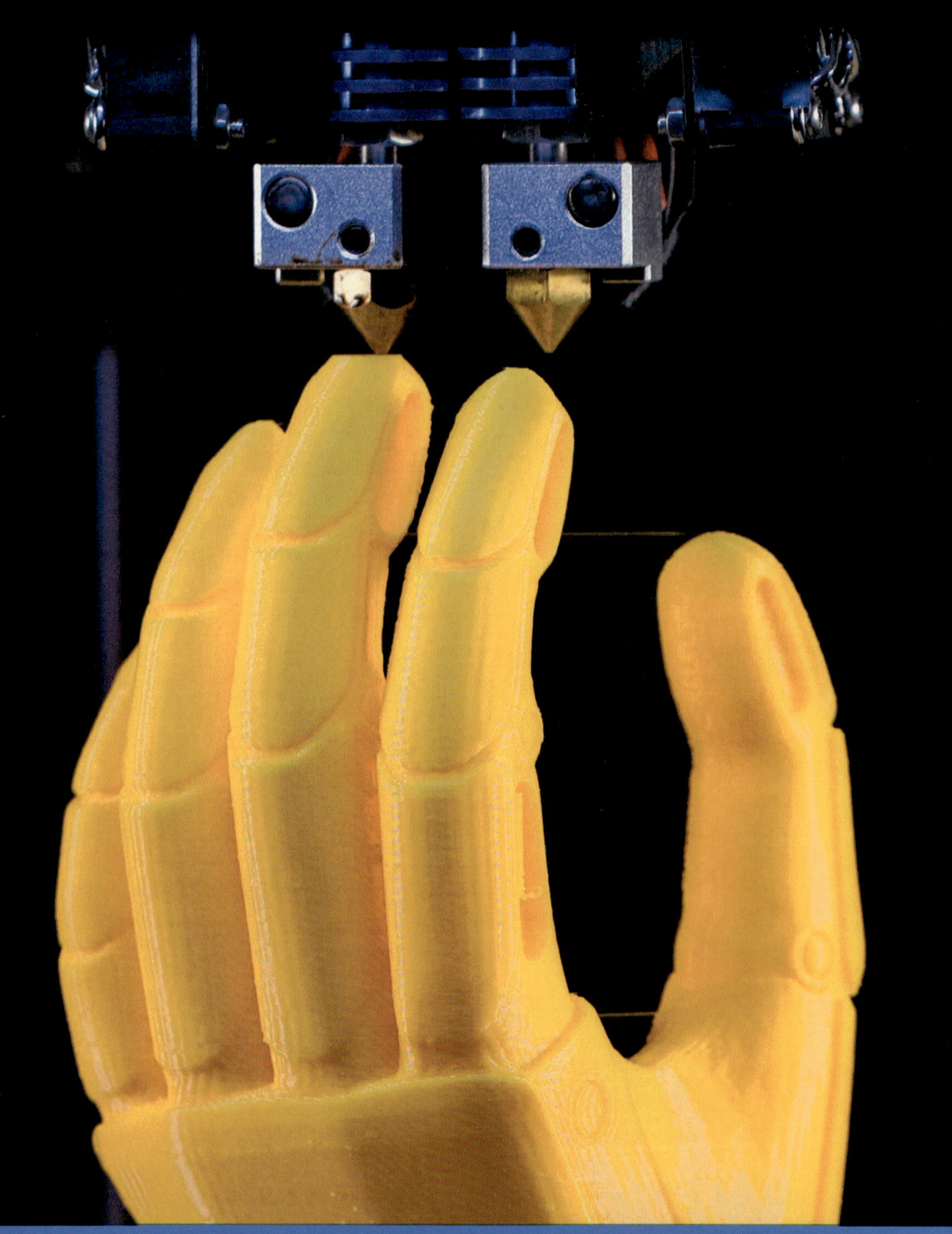
3D printing has many potential uses in health care.

the technology over time. Today companies print things such as plastic toys, silver jewelry, and metal machine parts.

Medical experts began using 3D printing for health care in the 1990s. Instead of plastic or metal, they use **biomaterials** or living **cells**. Printing human body parts is more difficult than printing a plastic toy. These parts need to work correctly with the rest of the body. Making this happen can be difficult. Scientists are working to improve 3D printing in health care to save lives.

CHAPTER ONE

WHAT IS THE HISTORY OF 3D PRINTING IN HEALTH CARE?

Charles Hull invented 3D printing in the 1980s. Hull is an engineer and a physics expert. He worked for a company in California. At the company, Hull used light to harden liquid plastic into strong, solid surfaces for tabletops. He came up with a

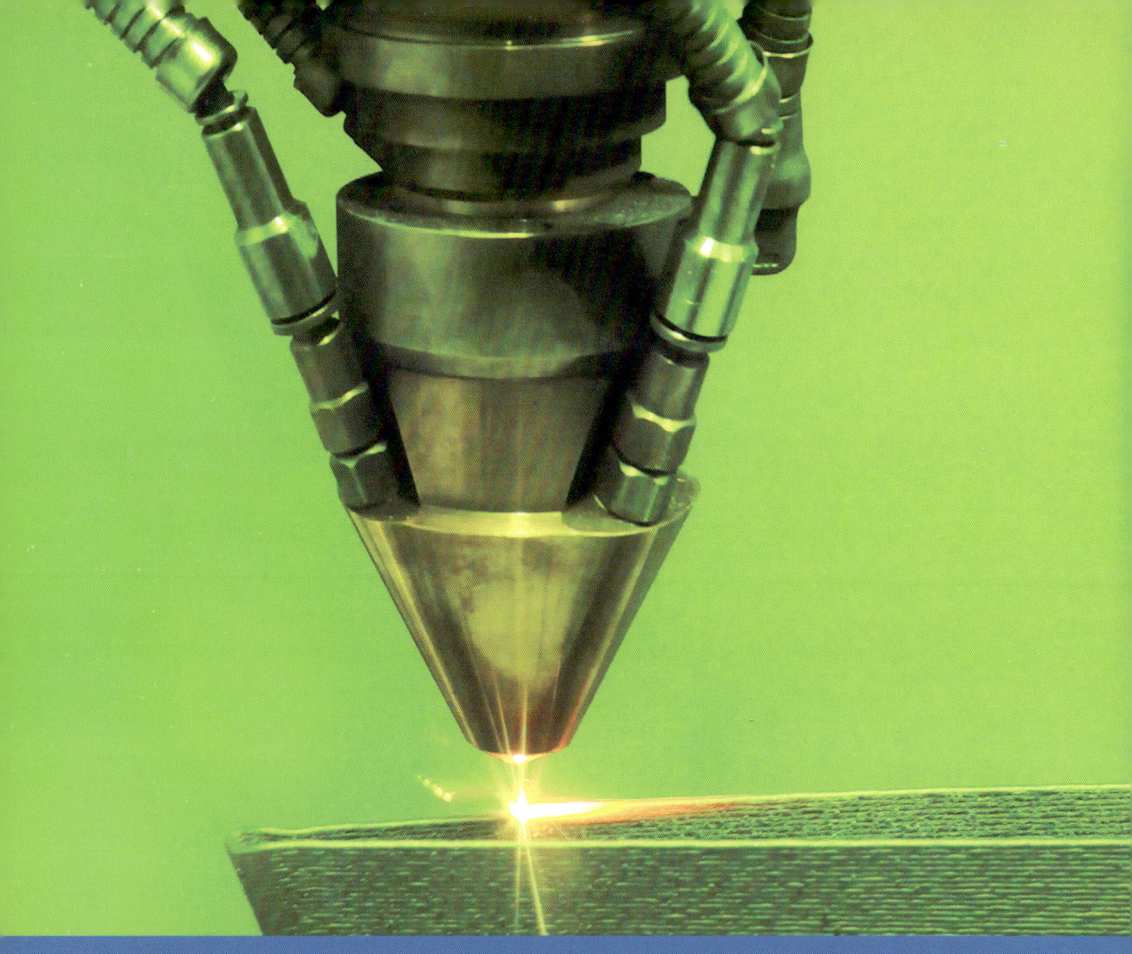

Many 3D printers today still use lasers.

new way to use this technology. First, he made a model of an object on a computer. This digital file was sent to a special printer. The printer used a **laser** to harden liquid plastic that was pushed out of a nozzle.

By hardening many layers of plastic, Hull could build up a 3D object. In 1983, he did this for the first time. He used his printer to make a small plastic knob. Hull called his process stereolithography.

In 1986, Hull started his own company, 3D Systems. By 1988, he was making and

ADDITIVE MANUFACTURING

Another name for 3D printing is additive manufacturing. Before 3D printing, objects were often made by removing rather than adding materials. A product might start as a block of wood or plastic. Parts are chopped or drilled away to create the product. The leftover material is waste. Since 3D printing adds only the material needed, there is less waste.

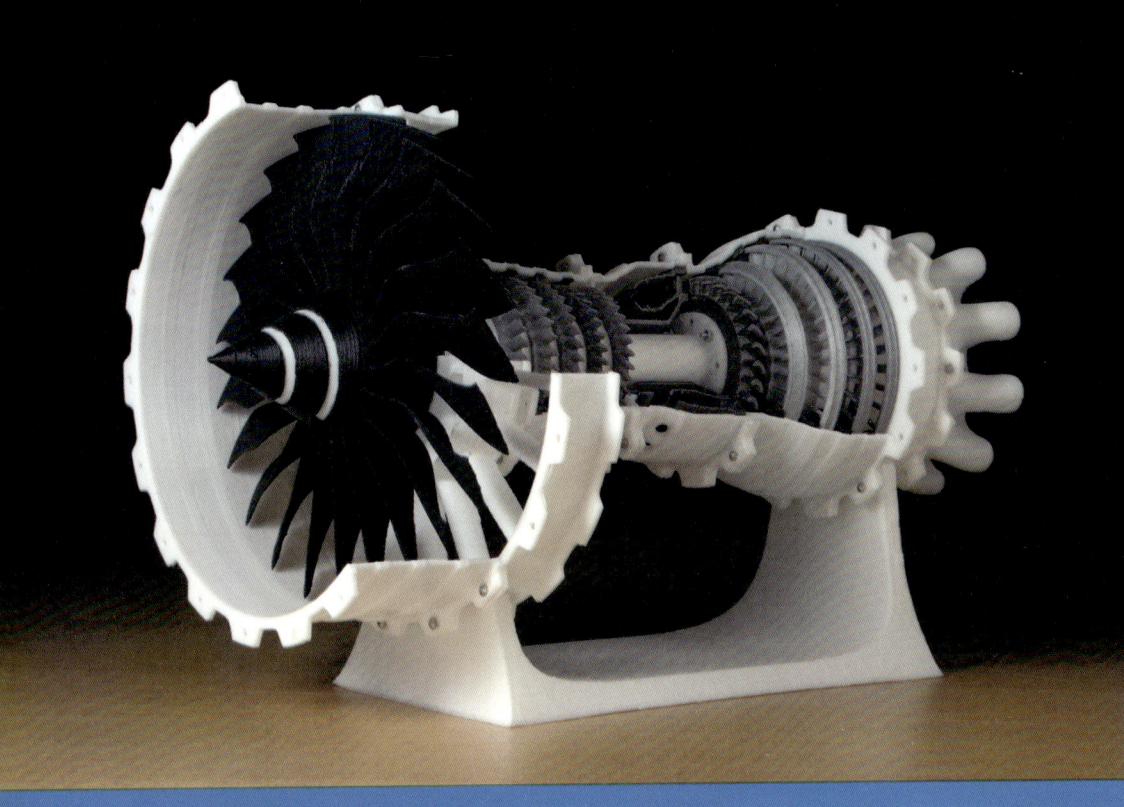

3D printing can be useful for making models of new airplane or car parts.

selling 3D printers. Car and airplane makers began using them to make models and molds of parts. At first, 3D printed parts weren't sturdy enough to last for long. But soon, inventors found stronger materials for 3D printing.

Hull didn't have medical uses in mind at first. But he later saw the potential. He told an interviewer, "To me, some of the medical applications [have been the most surprising]. I didn't anticipate that, and as soon as I started working with some of the medical imaging people, it became pretty clear that this was going to work."[1]

3D PRINTING FOR FUN

3D printers for home use are much simpler and cheaper than the ones scientists use. They can make nuts, bolts, eyeglasses, jewelry, toys, and even food. Schools and libraries use 3D printers in special areas called makerspaces. Hobbyists can get free designs for 3D objects online.

PRINTING TISSUES AND ORGANS

Tissues are groups of similar cells. They work together to do a certain job in the body. Groups of tissues make up organs. Organs include the kidney and the liver. Organs keep a person alive and healthy.

Biomaterials are materials that can work alongside living parts of the body. Scientists create biomaterials to repair or replace tissues that are injured. Making replacement tissues by hand is difficult. It takes a long time. It is expensive. In the 1990s, medical researchers wondered if they could use 3D printing to make tissues or even organs.

They could design a computer model of the object. Then they could build it with a special 3D printer. If everything worked right, the tissue or organ could be placed in a patient. It could keep the patient healthy.

Dr. Anthony Atala is the director of the Wake Forest Institute for Regenerative Medicine (WFIRM) in Winston-Salem, North Carolina. In 1999, he and his team used a 3D printer to form biomaterials into the shape of a human bladder. They coated this object with live human bladder cells. The cells grew and formed a pouch. Atala put these pouches around the bladders

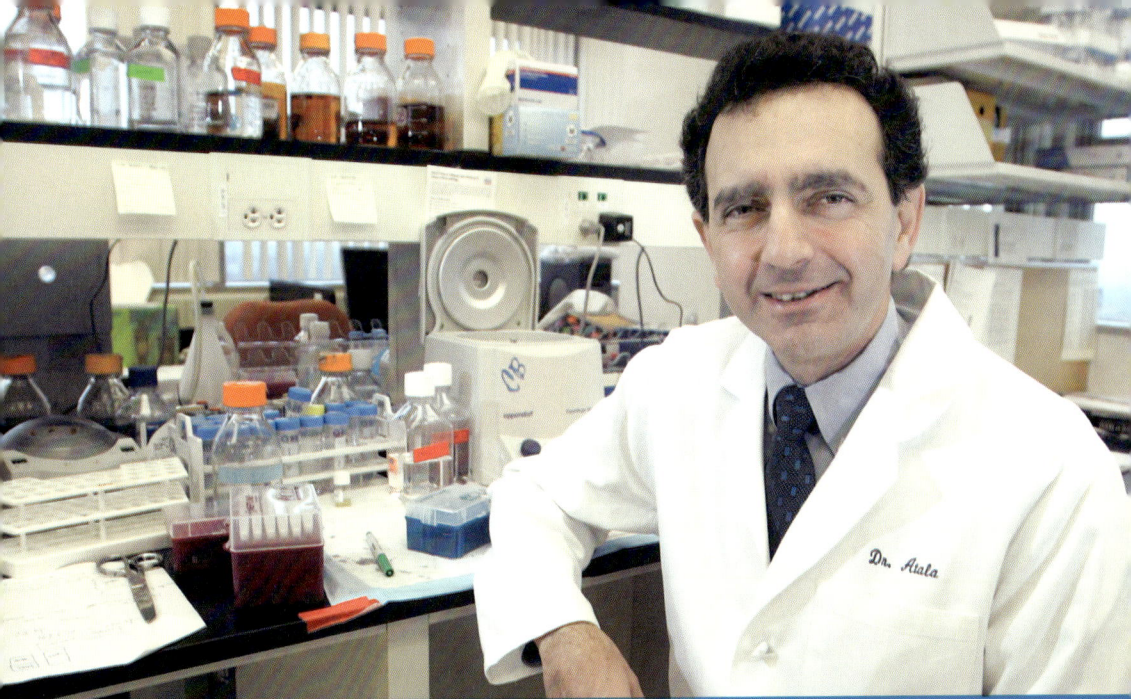

Anthony Atala has been a pioneer in 3D printing human tissue.

of seven children whose bladders did not work. The operations were successful.

Atala's work pioneered 3D printing in health care. Atala says, "Back in the '90s we created by hand, even without using the printer, bladders, skin, cartilage . . . and later implanted them successfully in patients. The printer automated what we were already doing and scaled it up, making some of the processes easier."[2]

3D BIOPRINTING

Dr. Thomas Boland is a biomedical engineer. In 2000, he had the idea to try printing with living cells. Boland tested his idea with an inkjet printer. This is the kind of printer many people have at home. It sprays tiny jets of ink to print words and pictures.

Boland replaced the printer's ink with collagen, a protein found in skin. He glued a thin sheet of black silicon onto a sheet of paper and put it in the printer. Then

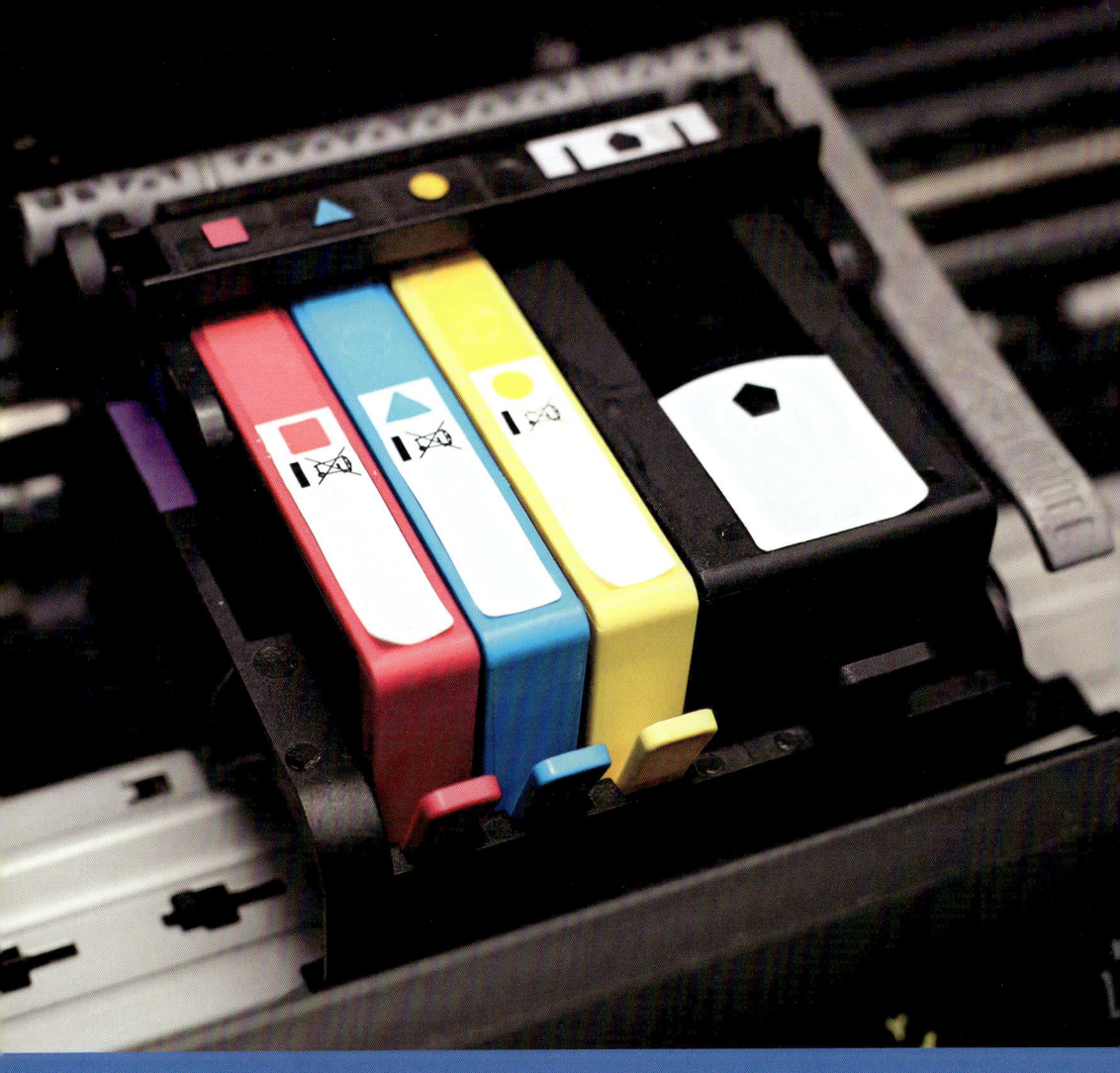

Inkjet printers use cartridges containing ink of different colors. Boland replaced the ink with collagen for his experiments.

he typed his initials into a program on his

computer and hit the print command. It

worked. The paper came out showing "TB"

in off-white collagen. This was the start of bioprinting.

Boland and his team went on to print with bacteria. They also used cells from hamsters and rats. After printing, 90 percent of the cells they used stayed alive. This showed that the process could be useful for health care.

At first Boland printed live cells in one layer. Next, he added a platform to his printer. After each layer was printed, the platform lowered. The printer laid down the next layer of cells. Now Boland was 3D bioprinting. This was a big breakthrough.

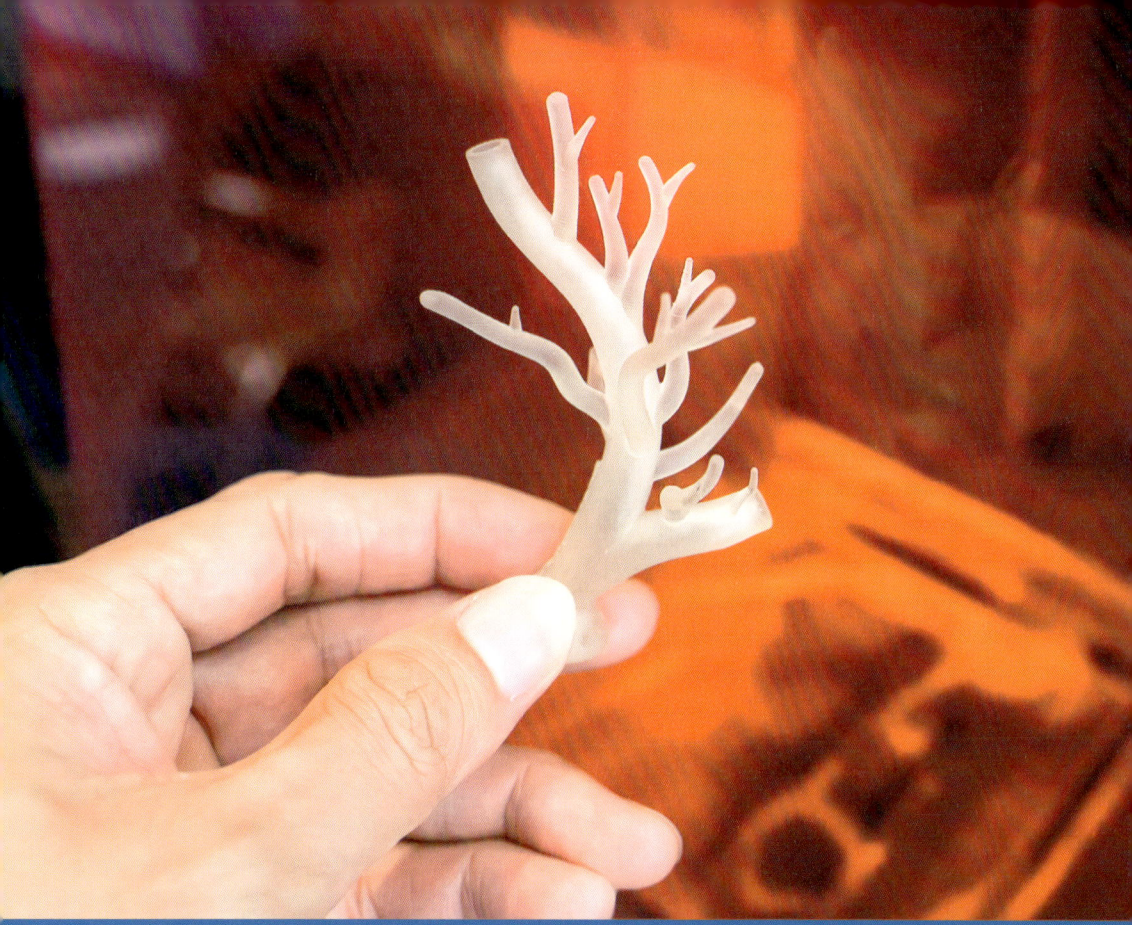

Printing blood vessels is a major area of research.

CONTINUED BREAKTHROUGHS

In 2008, the first 3D printed prosthetic leg was given to a patient. By 2010, a bioprinting company in San Diego, California, had printed the first blood vessel.

It began testing them in animals before human use could begin.

New advances came from around the world. In 2015, a company in Sweden called Cellink demonstrated an ink made from seaweed. It could be used to print cartilage, a connective tissue found in the human body. In 2019, Israeli scientists made the first 3D printed heart using human cells. The heart didn't beat, and it was too small for human use. But it could be used to help scientists understand how to make a working human heart in the future.

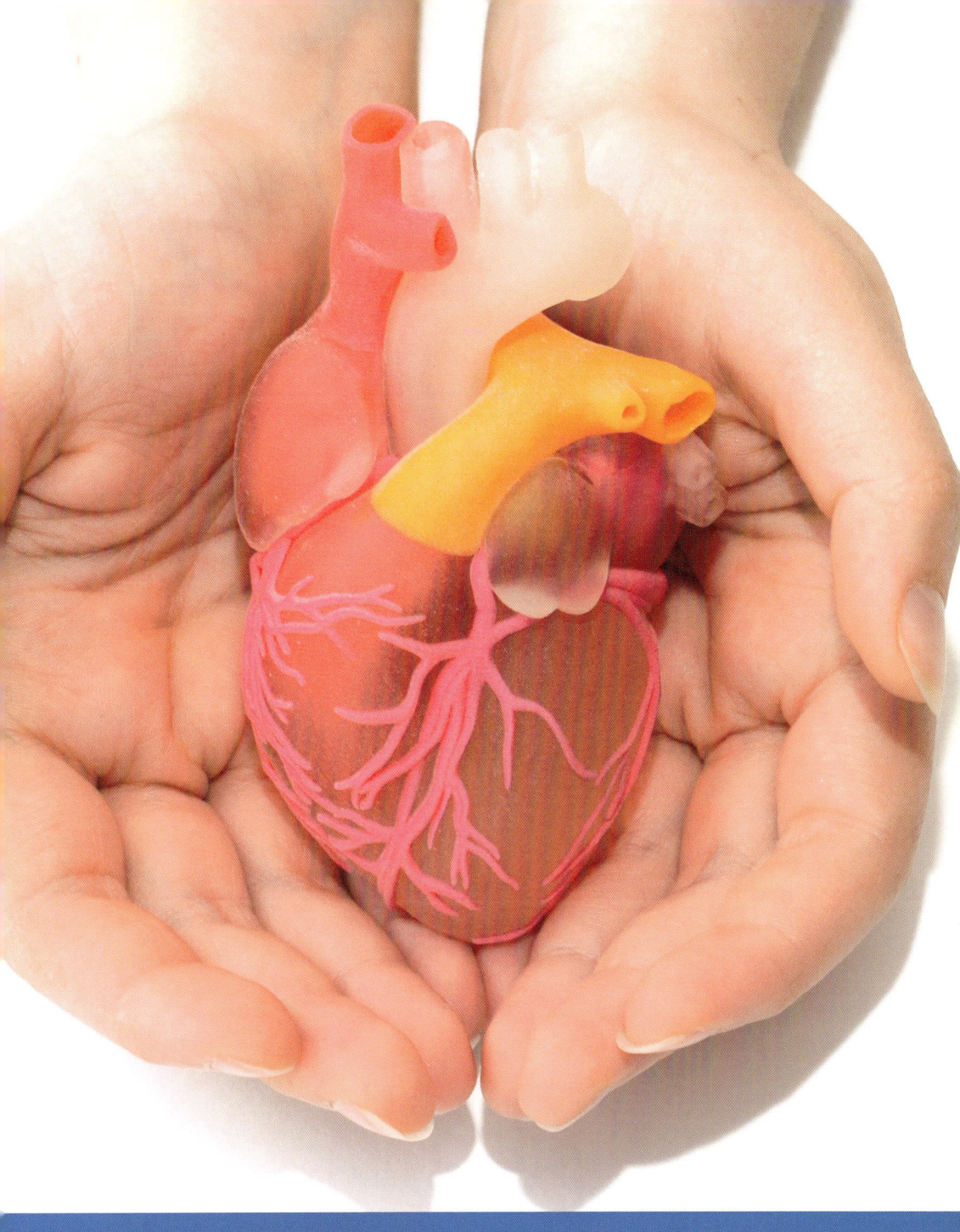

A functioning 3D printed heart would be a major breakthrough.

CHAPTER TWO

HOW DOES 3D PRINTING IN HEALTH CARE WORK?

3D printers that create objects using plastic or metal can be used in health care. These work similarly to 3D printers used in education, engineering, and other fields. But one type of 3D printing is unique to health care. It is called bioprinting.

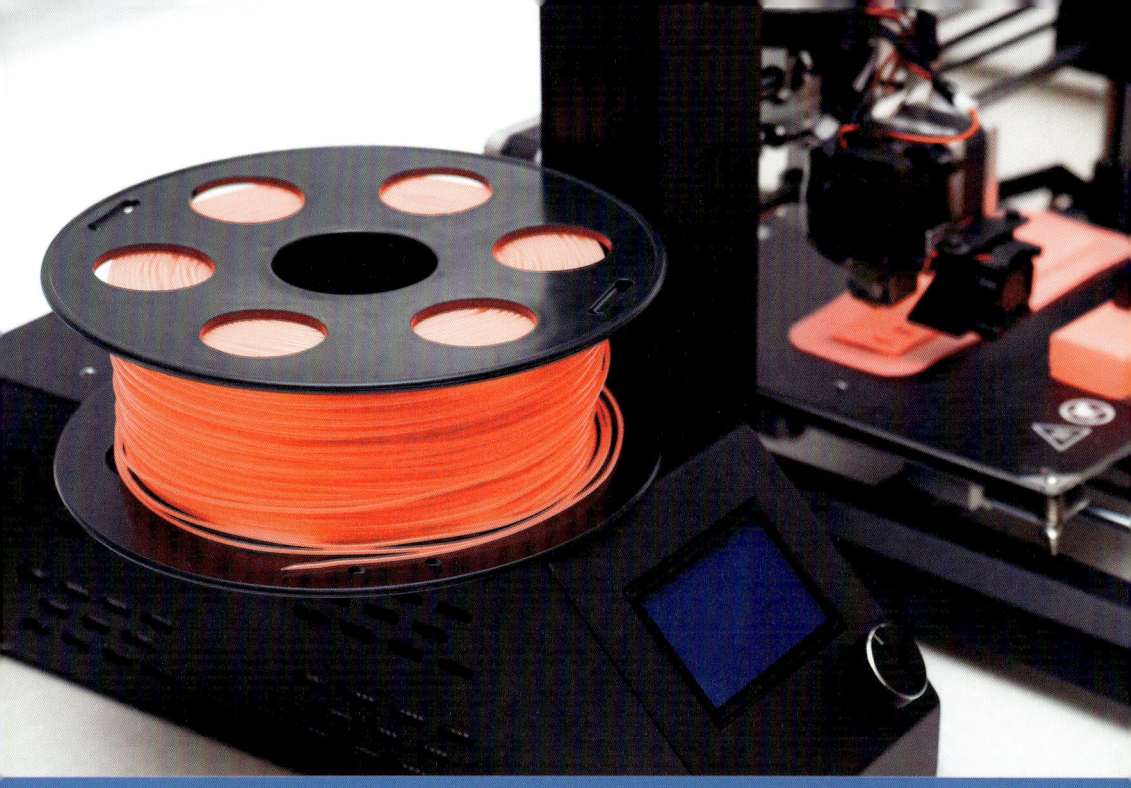

Home 3D printers often use plastic materials called filament to print. Bioprinters use living cells instead.

Bioprinting prints with living cells. These biomaterials are known as bioink. The devices that use these materials are called bioprinters. This type of printing allows doctors to create parts that can be used inside the human body. Scientists use bioprinters to make tissue, bone, or other body parts for patients.

Human tissues and organs are more complex than plastic toys or metal machine parts. They must work with a network of other body parts. They connect to blood vessels. This is how tissues and organs get the oxygen that keeps them alive.

LETTING CELLS DO THE WORK

Inside the body, cells can adapt to change the structures they make up. Researchers found that bioprinted cells do the same thing. After printing a blood vessel, they saw that the cells worked to strengthen the blood vessel. They even began forming tiny new blood vessels on the end of the structure.

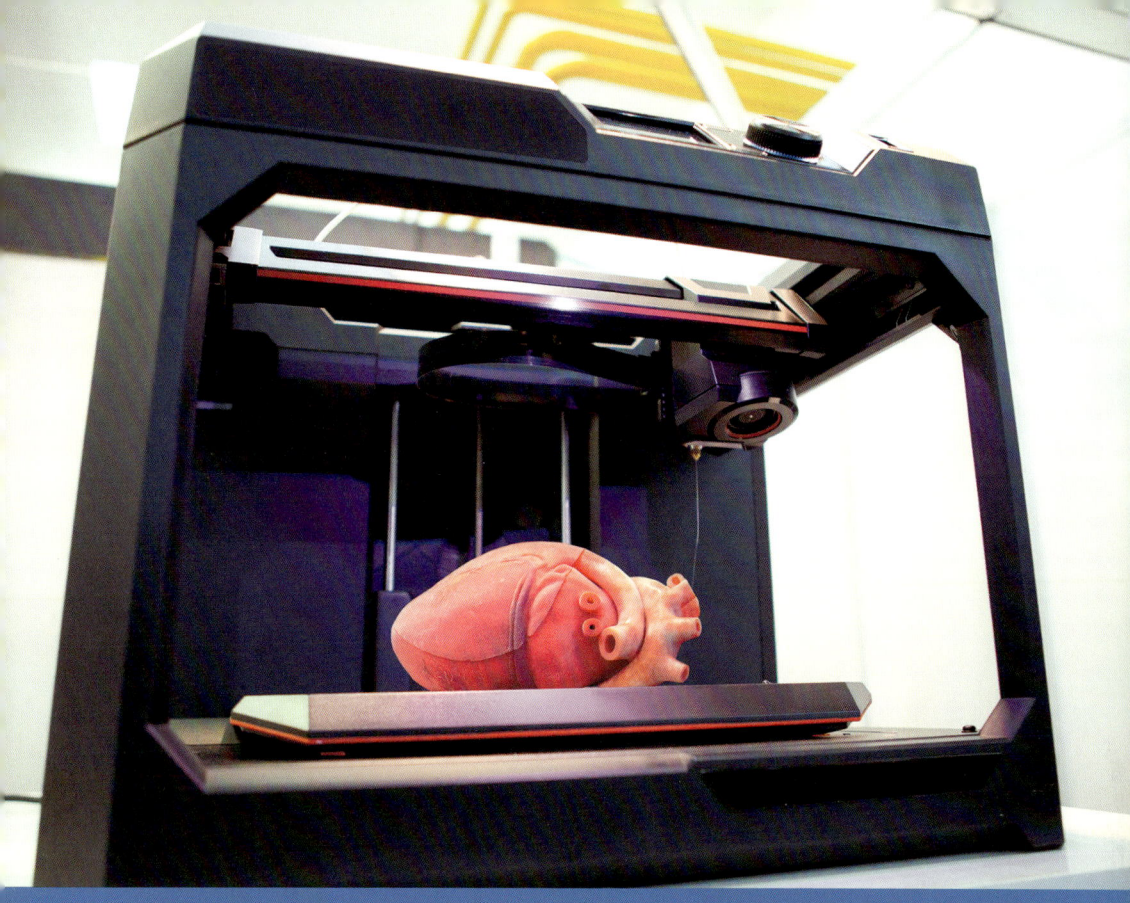

Bioprinting could one day let scientists print working organs.

Researchers are learning how to make these connections work.

BIOPRINTER TYPES AND PARTS

There are four types of bioprinters. Inkjet printers send bioink through tiny nozzles

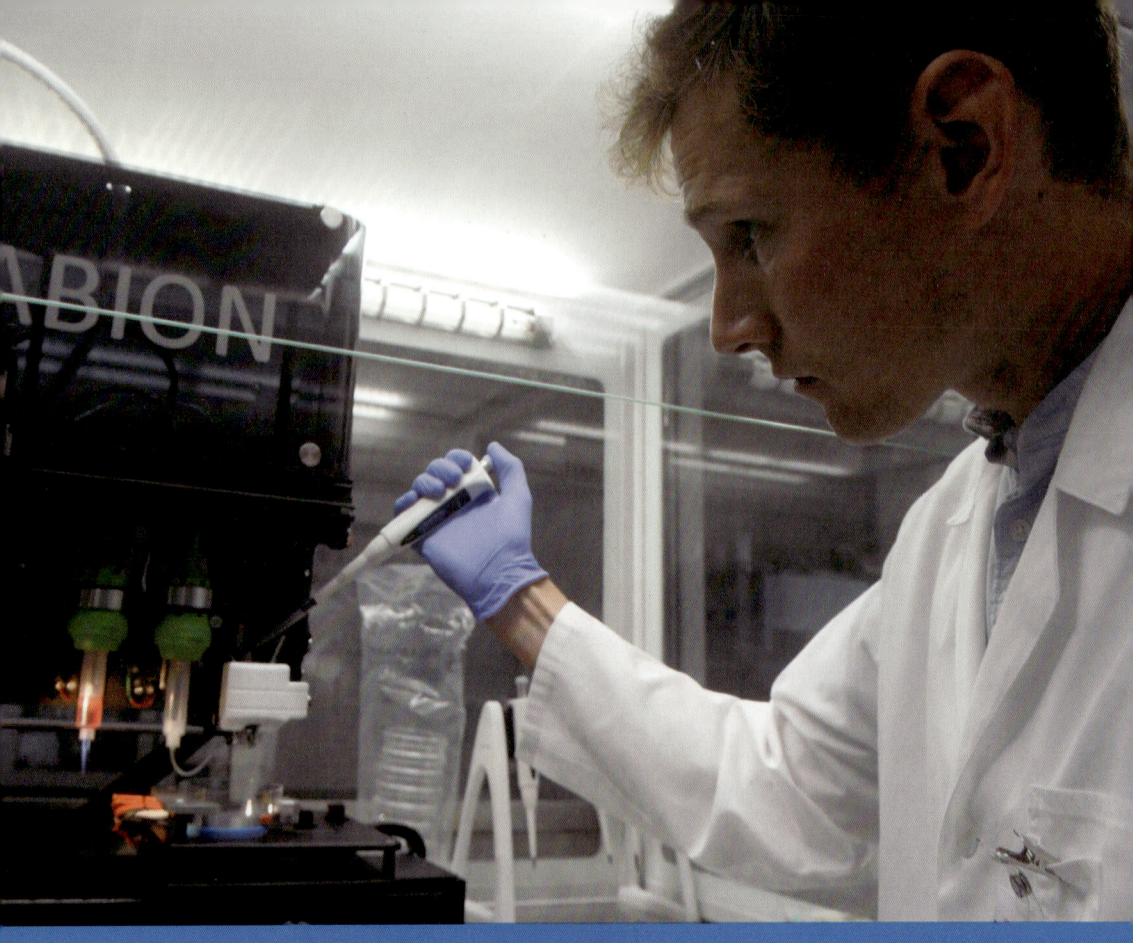

A researcher works with a 3D bioprinter.

with heat or vibration. Laser printers use a laser beam to dispense bioink. Extrusion printers force the bioink out with pressure. Electrospray or electrospin printers use electric fields to push out the bioink.

The different types of bioprinters have different uses. Inkjet printers are the cheapest type. But bioink that is too thick or sticky does not work well in an inkjet printer. The other types of printers can handle those bioinks. They can print more complex shapes. But heat from the laser can damage the bioink. So can pressure from extrusion printers and electricity from electrospray or electrospin printers.

Bioprinters generally contain a few key parts. A **reservoir** holds the bioink. It is connected to the print head, where the bioink comes out. Motors move the print

3D BIOPRINTER PARTS

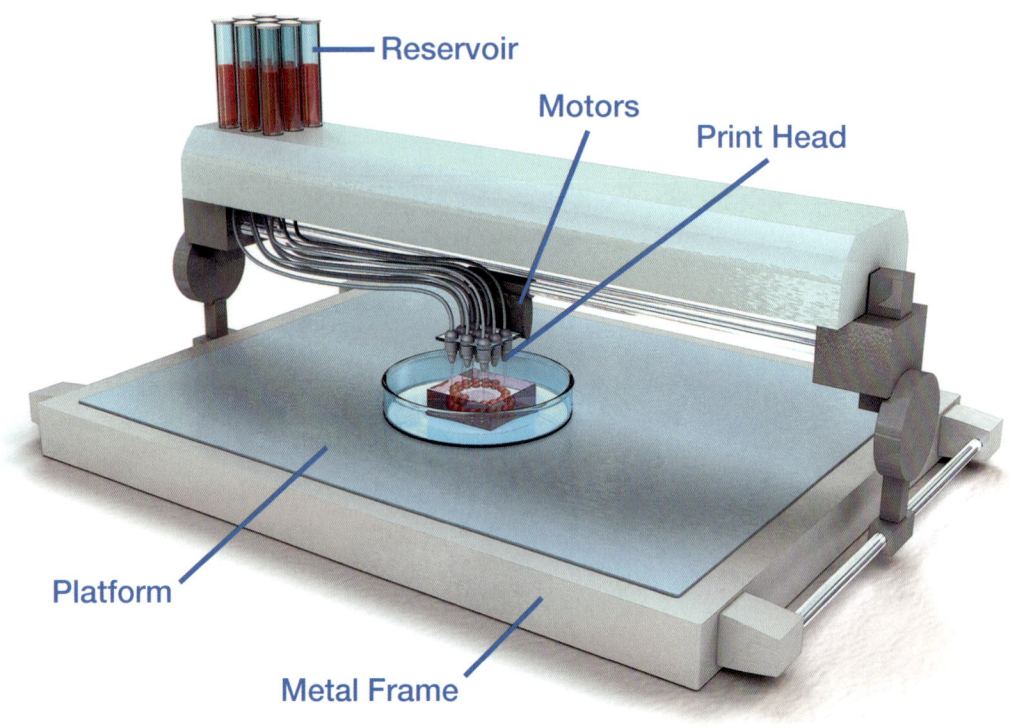

3D bioprinters come in different shapes and sizes, but they share many basic parts.

head around during printing. The object being printed sits on a platform. Another set of motors shifts the platform around as needed. All these parts are supported by a large metal frame.

BIOPRINTING STEP-BY-STEP

Doctors follow a series of steps to bioprint body parts. First, they need to make a plan for the part to be printed. This is similar to the way an architect draws a plan for a building. To make the plan, the doctor may start with a medical scan. Devices called CT scanners or MRI scanners create images of the inside of a patient's body. They take pictures of tissues, blood vessels, or organs.

The scanner sends those images to a computer. The doctor can turn them into a digital three-dimensional model. Computer software splits that model up into layers. It creates instructions for the 3D printer. It tells the printer how to build the body part.

CT AND MRI SCANS

A computerized tomography (CT) scan uses X-ray images taken from different angles. It creates computer images of bones, blood vessels, or soft tissues inside a body. Magnetic resonance imaging (MRI) uses a magnetic field and radio waves to take images inside the body.

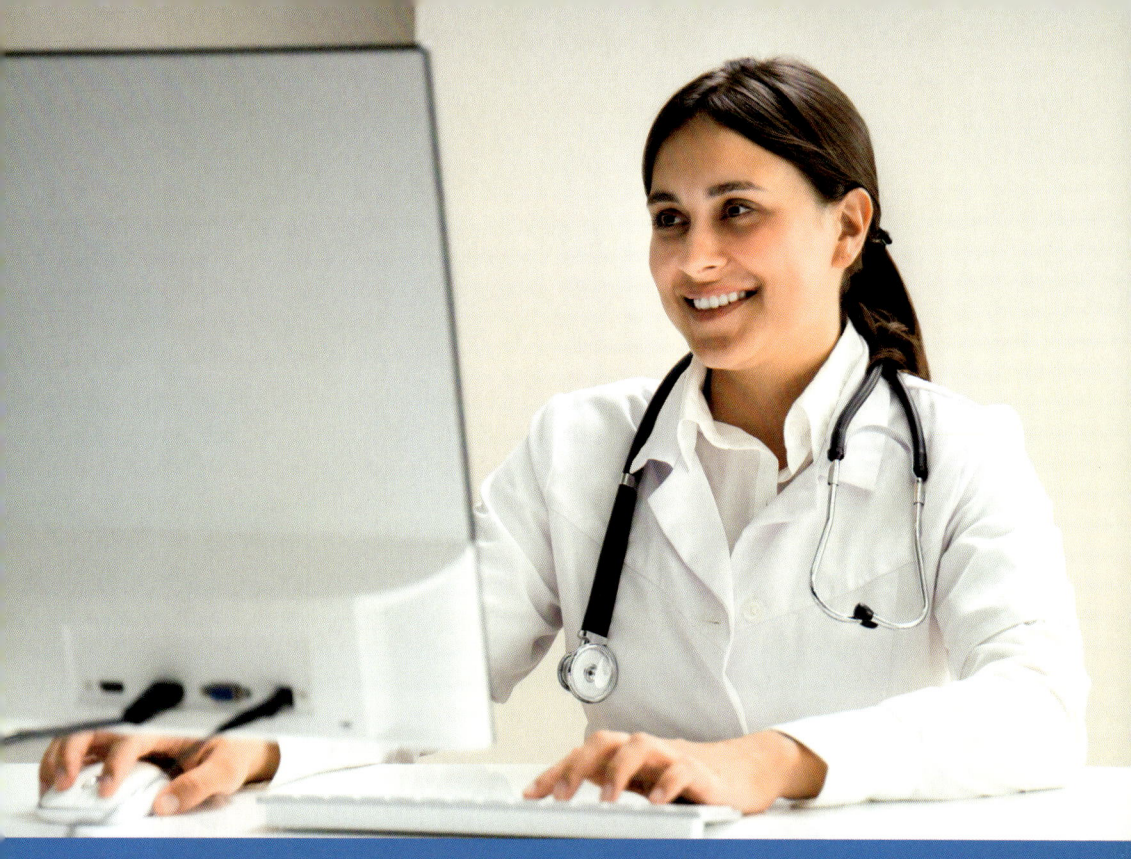

Doctors use computers to create 3D models of objects they need to print.

Next a scientist prepares the bioink. She takes living cells from the patient. She adds them to a base made of materials such as collagen. The base gives the cells a structure to sit on and a place to grow.

37

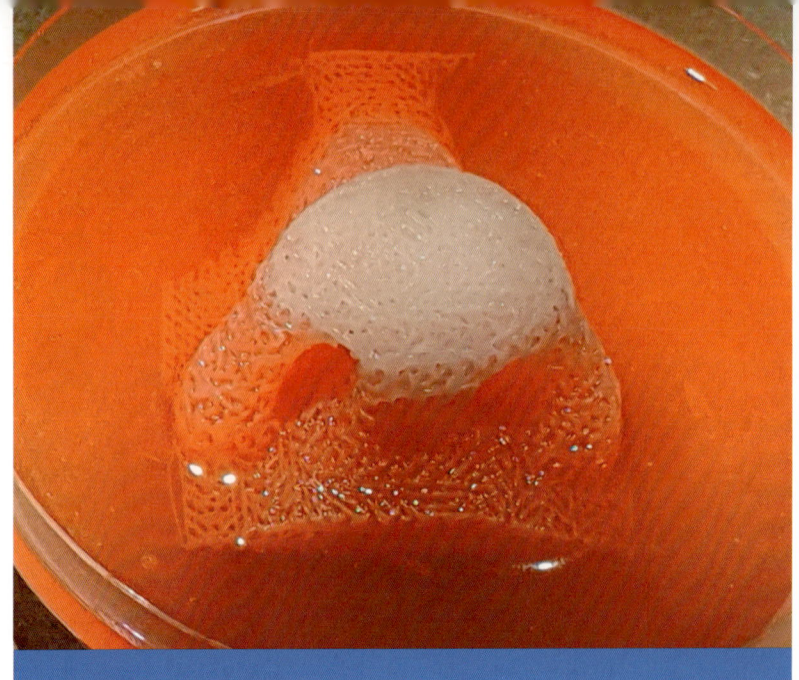

A 3D bioprinted nose

The base material also provides water and **nutrients** to the cells.

The bioink is loaded into the printer's reservoir, and the printer starts to work. It prints the body part layer by layer. Bioprinters may use light, chemicals, or heat to help the printed shape become solid and hold its shape. After printing, the doctor places the body part in an incubator. This is a closed container that keeps it warm. Here the cells in the tissue start to work together. The tissue can be implanted in a patient.

The process works similarly for bioprinted organs. Experts have made organs that stay alive in an incubator for up to forty days. They have not yet printed organs that can be implanted in humans. But experts continue to work toward that goal. Jennifer Lewis is a professor of engineering. She spoke about the possibility of printing working organs. "It's exciting," she said, "but there's still more work to be done."[3]

CHAPTER THREE

HOW ARE DOCTORS USING 3D PRINTING TODAY?

A human body part is very complex. Different types of cells and tissues need to work together. Cells and tissues come together to form organs. All these parts must function correctly for a person to live. Because a body is alive, each part

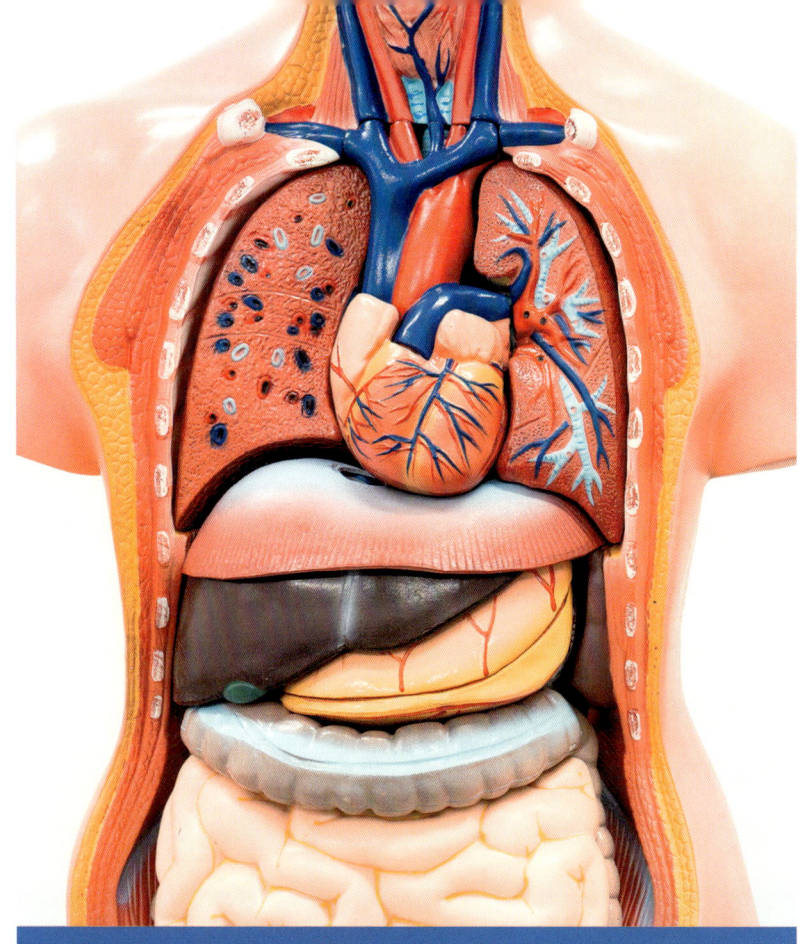

The human body is made up of many complex parts. These parts must work together properly to keep a person alive and healthy.

also needs nutrients. Making all this happen with **artificial** parts is challenging. It makes bioprinting more difficult than other kinds of 3D printing.

Medical experts have been working on these problems since the 1990s. They have made many big advances. Doctors are now using 3D printing in many ways. They can make tissues to put in the body. They can build custom artificial limbs and joints. They can even use 3D printing to research new drugs.

BIOPRINTING TISSUES

Dr. Atala and his team at WFIRM are experienced with tissues. They have been implanting tissues made from his patients' cells since the 1990s. They began using

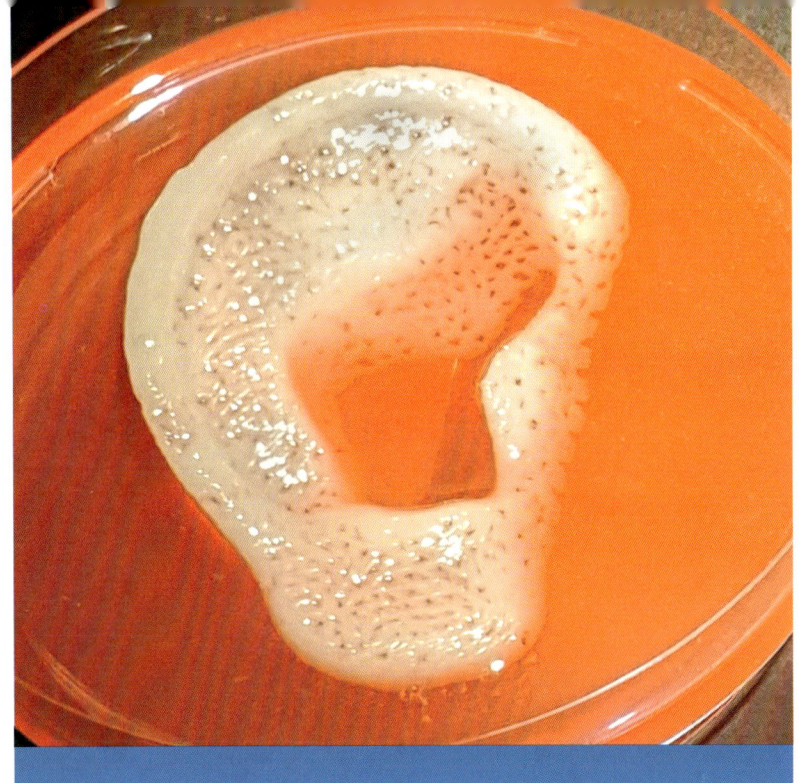

An ear printed by the team at WFIRM

3D bioprinting in the late 1990s. They continue to make advances in this area.

Doctors have created 3D printed ears. They are made of cartilage. These parts can be given to a patient with a damaged ear. First, doctors scan the patient's healthy ear.

They use this data to design a new ear.
Then they print a mold of the ear. The
doctors add cartilage cells and collagen.
They let the ear grow in an incubator. Then
they attach it to the patient.

PRINTING JOINTS AND BONES

3D printing can also help people with joint

problems. Joints are the parts of the body

ORGANS

Some human tissues are simpler than others. This makes them easier to 3D print. Organs that are flat like the skin or hollow like the bladder are less complex. Organs like the heart, liver, or kidney have more cells. They also have more types of cells. This makes them trickier to 3D print.

where two bones connect. Knees and hips are examples of joints. Orthopedists are doctors who work with bones and joints. Many patients have worn or injured joints. Orthopedists can replace them with 3D printed joints.

Daniel Wiznia of Yale University works in this area. He explains that 3D printing is useful for joints. He says, "Everyone's anatomy is unique, which means the shape of your bone is going to be different from the shape of someone else's. So, you would want implants made specifically for you."[4]

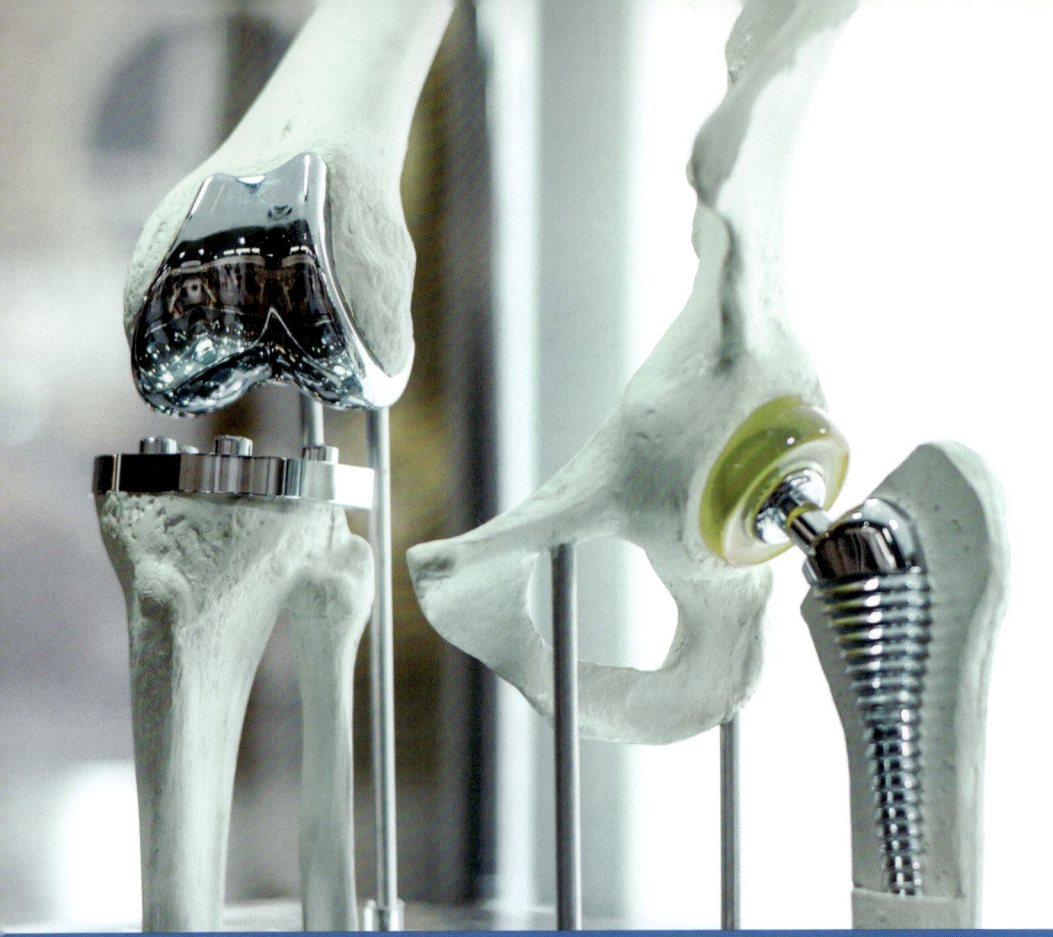

Artificial knee and hip joints improve many patients' lives. 3D printing can make these devices even better.

Orthopedists might use plastic, ceramic, or **titanium** as printing materials. The joint is made to be strong. But it is also **porous**. This allows the patient's bones to grow into the surface of the joint after surgery. This creates a stronger connection.

Printed bones can be used elsewhere in the body too. Doctors in the Netherlands created a lower jaw bone on a 3D printer. They used titanium powder as the material. The printer used a laser to heat the powder. This formed a hard structure. It took thousands of layers to finish the jaw. The doctors replaced a patient's infected jaw with the 3D printed bone.

Patients sometimes have damaged or diseased bones. They commonly need bone grafts to repair the bones. In a bone

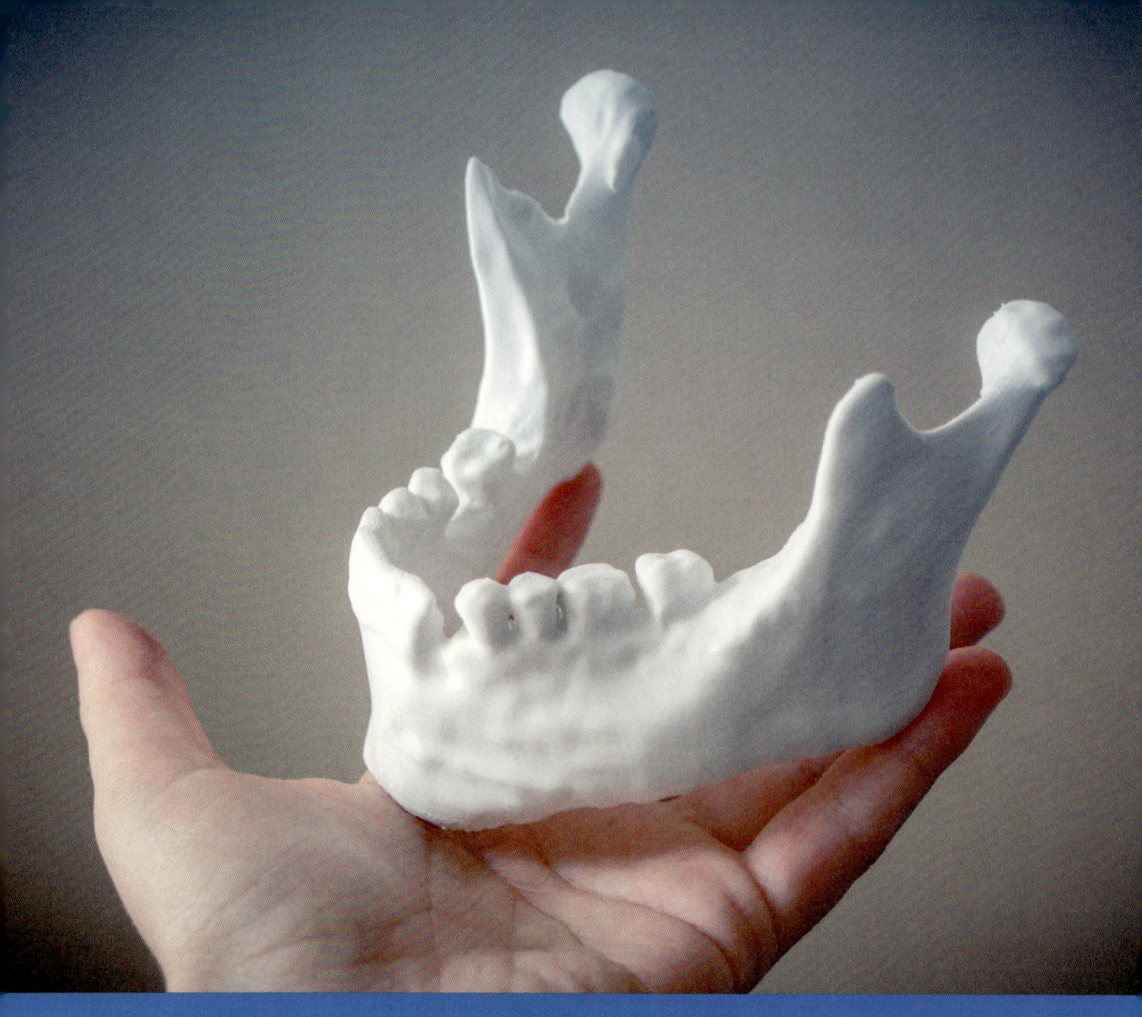

Doctors are studying the possibilities of 3D printed bones.

graft, doctors join nonliving material to a patient's bone. A team of Australian doctors developed a way to use 3D printing for bone grafts. They print an artificial bone that is placed into the body during surgery. Over several months, new bone grows over the implant. Eventually this new growth replaces the implanted bone.

OTHER MEDICAL PRODUCTS

3D printing is also a useful tool for making prosthetics. Prosthetics are artificial versions of body parts. They include arms, legs, hands, and other parts. Prosthetics have been in use for a long time. But 3D printing offers ways to improve them.

With 3D printing, doctors can make prosthetics with a custom fit. They can match the patient's body exactly. This

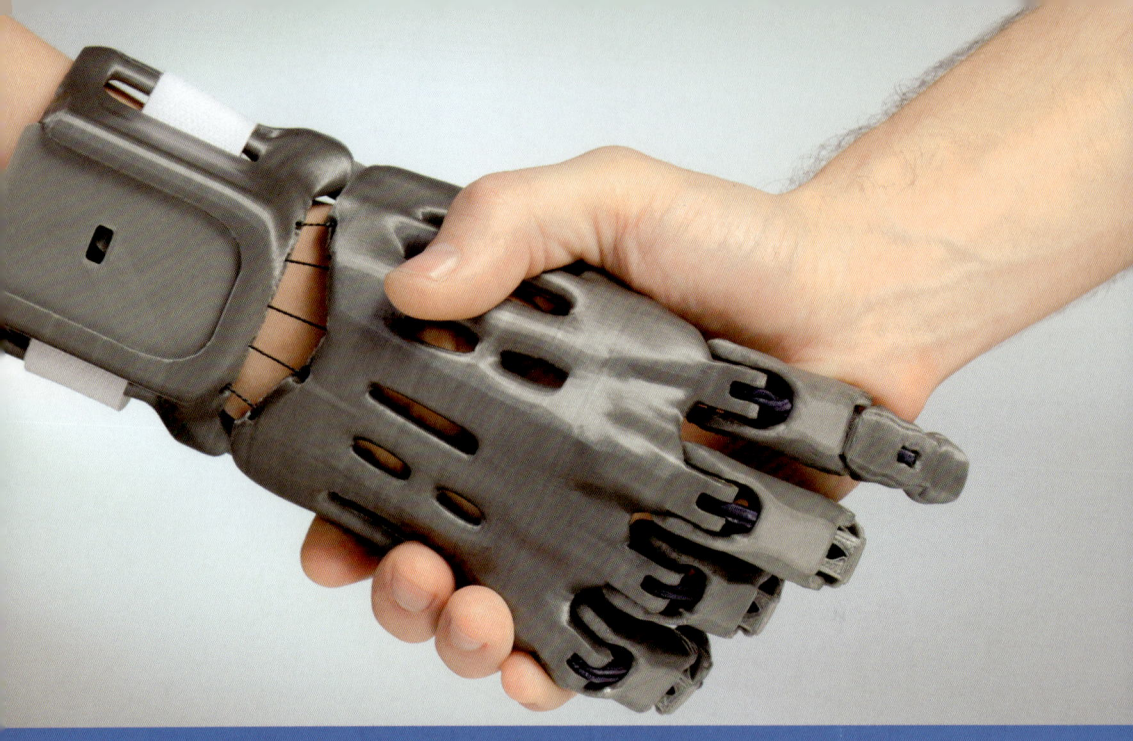

3D printing has a lot of potential for custom-fit prosthetics.

makes the prosthetics more comfortable. It also lets them work better. This is especially helpful for children who are growing. Doctors can 3D print new limbs for kids as they outgrow them. The prostheses fit better. They also cost less to make.

A custom fit is important for many other medical products too. Hearing aids are one example. Each person's ear canal is shaped differently. Many of today's hearing aids are 3D printed. A custom fit helps with braces too. Orthodontists are now 3D printing clear, removable plastic braces. They are custom made to fit each patient's teeth.

3D PRINTED CASTS

Doctors can now 3D print light, flexible casts to help patients heal broken bones. These casts are custom fit to each patient. They are waterproof and can be removed. They are more comfortable than traditional plaster casts.

EDUCATION AND DRUG DEVELOPMENT

3D printing can help patients directly. Doctors can print tissues and bones. But they can use 3D printing in other ways too. One example is in education. Medical schools use 3D printers to make models of organs. Then students can study how these organs work. They can practice surgery on realistic hearts, livers, and other structures.

Experienced surgeons can use this technology too. They can use 3D printing to make an organ, tissue, or bone that matches the patient's. They can use this printed object to practice the surgery.

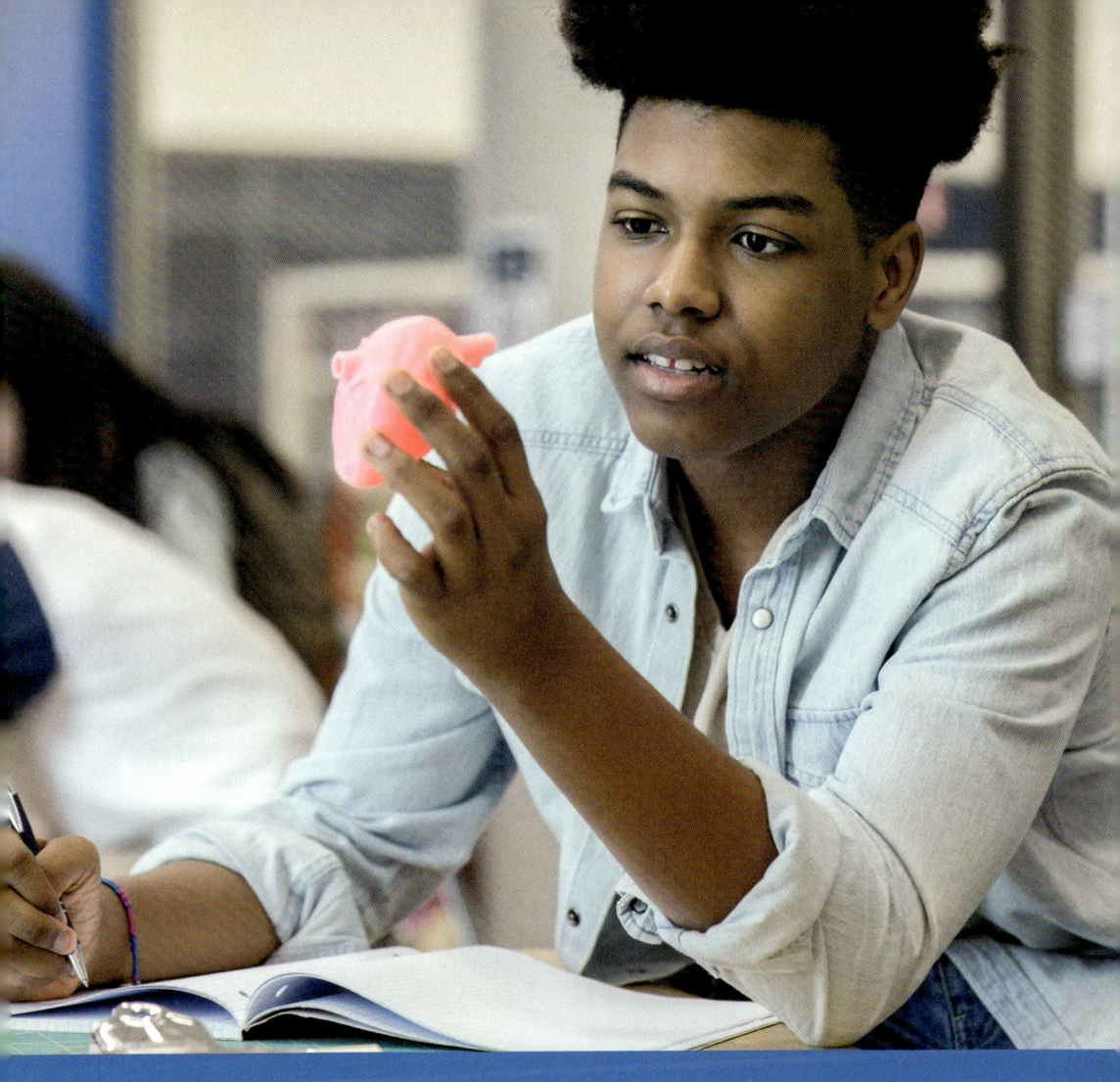

3D printed models of organs can be very useful in education.

This can improve the chances of success. It also prepares the surgeon to operate more quickly. This improves safety.

3D printing can even play a role in creating new drugs. Scientists can use 3D printed tissues and organs in testing. For example, the company Organovo prints models of liver, kidney, and cancer tissues. The tissue samples are kept alive in a lab. Scientists can test new drugs on these tissues. They can see how well the medicines work. It can be dangerous to test new drugs on live subjects. By using 3D printed tissue instead, researchers can avoid harming people or animals.

Drugmakers also use 3D printers to produce pills. Patients might need to take

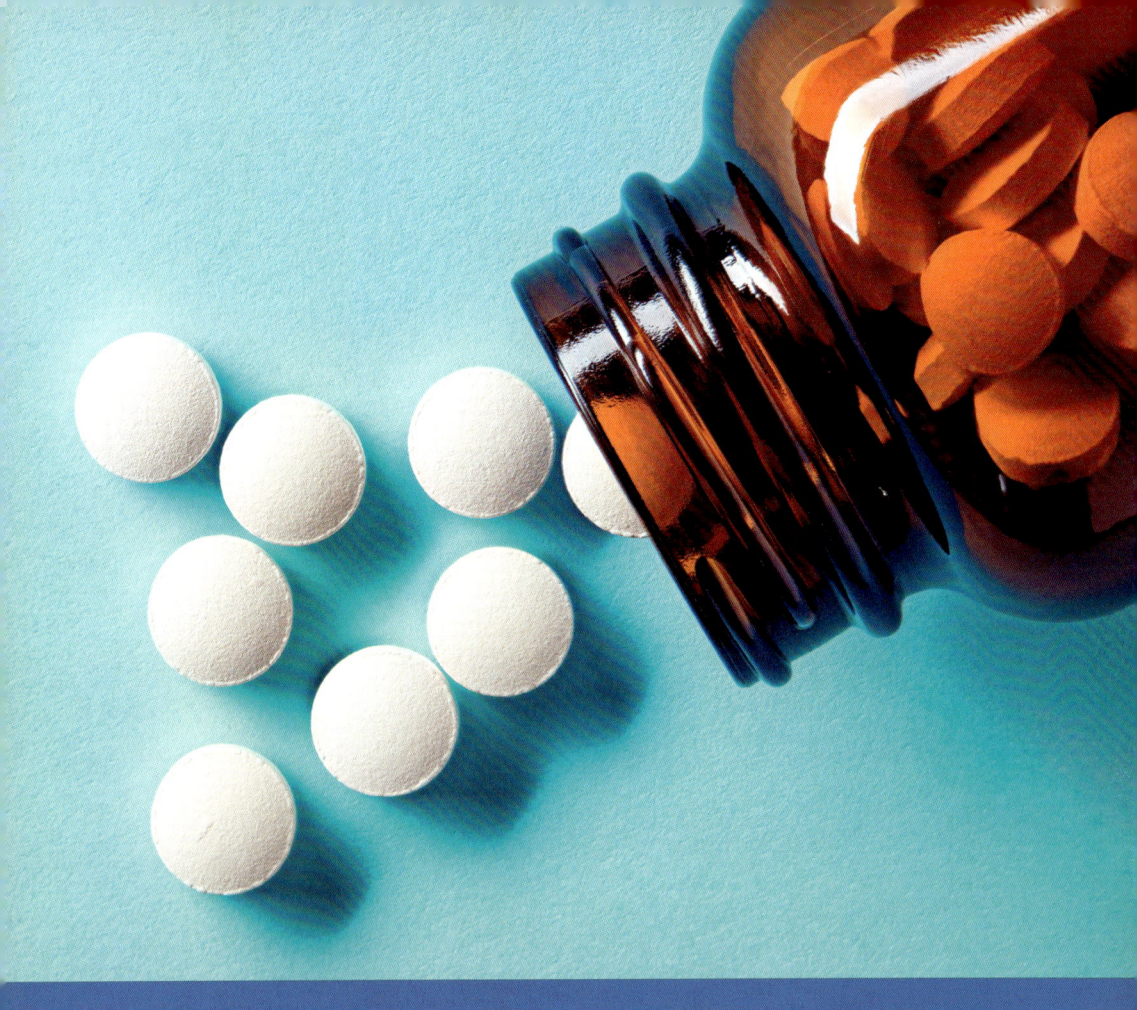

Doctors can use 3D printers to create custom pills containing the medicines each patient needs.

several different medicines. They might

need an amount that doesn't match the

standard pill dosage. In the past, patients

had to cut up pills themselves. Now experts

can print pills with just the right amount of medicine.

3D PRINTING AND COVID-19

The disease COVID-19 spread around the world in 2020. It was a deadly pandemic. More than 100 million people got sick. More than 2 million people died. The medical world worked to stop the pandemic. 3D printing played a role in this effort.

The virus that causes COVID-19 spreads through the air. It leaves the mouth or nose in tiny droplets. If other people contact these droplets, they can become sick. Doctors recommended that people use

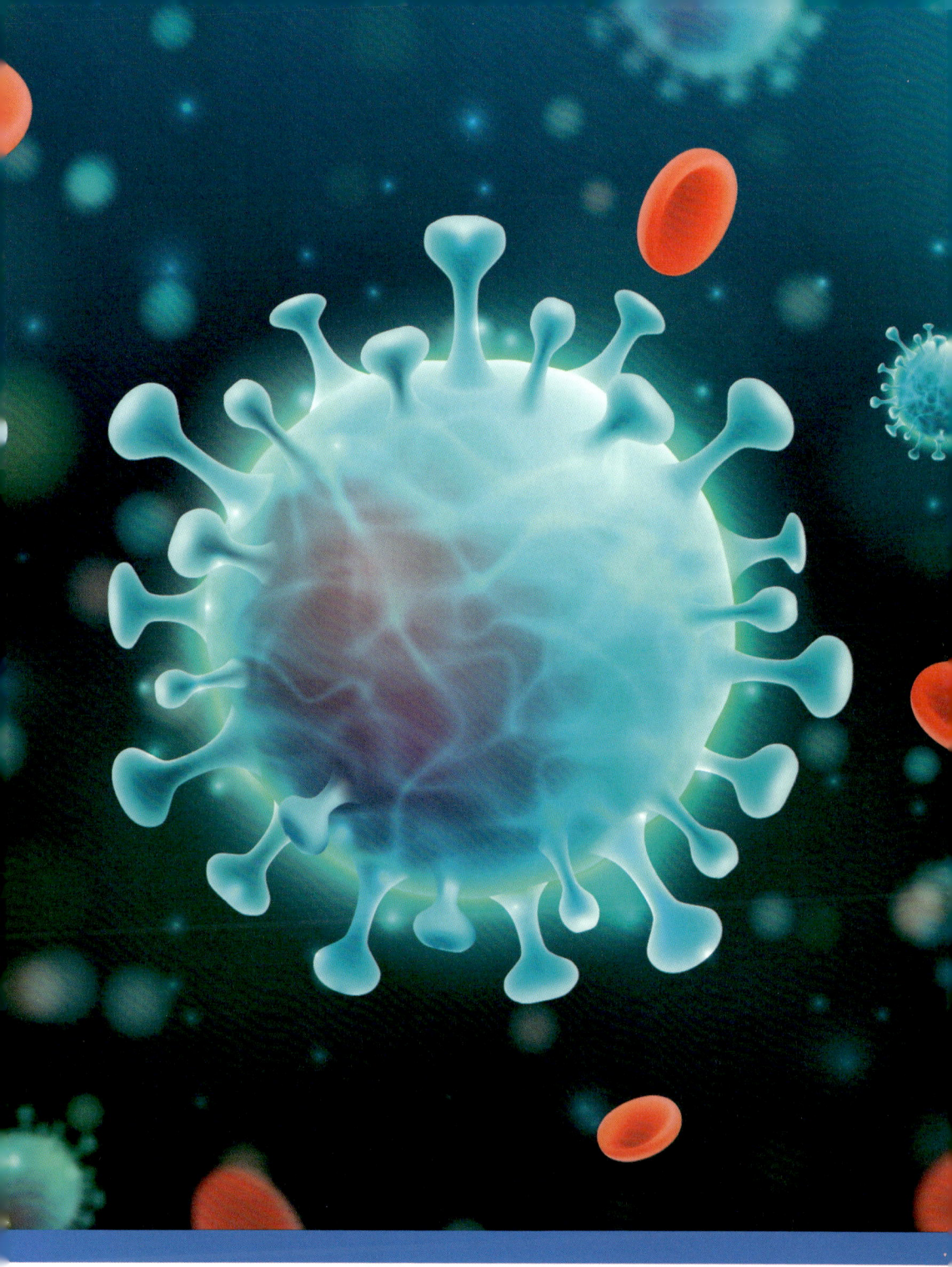

COVID-19 is caused by a virus called SARS-CoV-2.

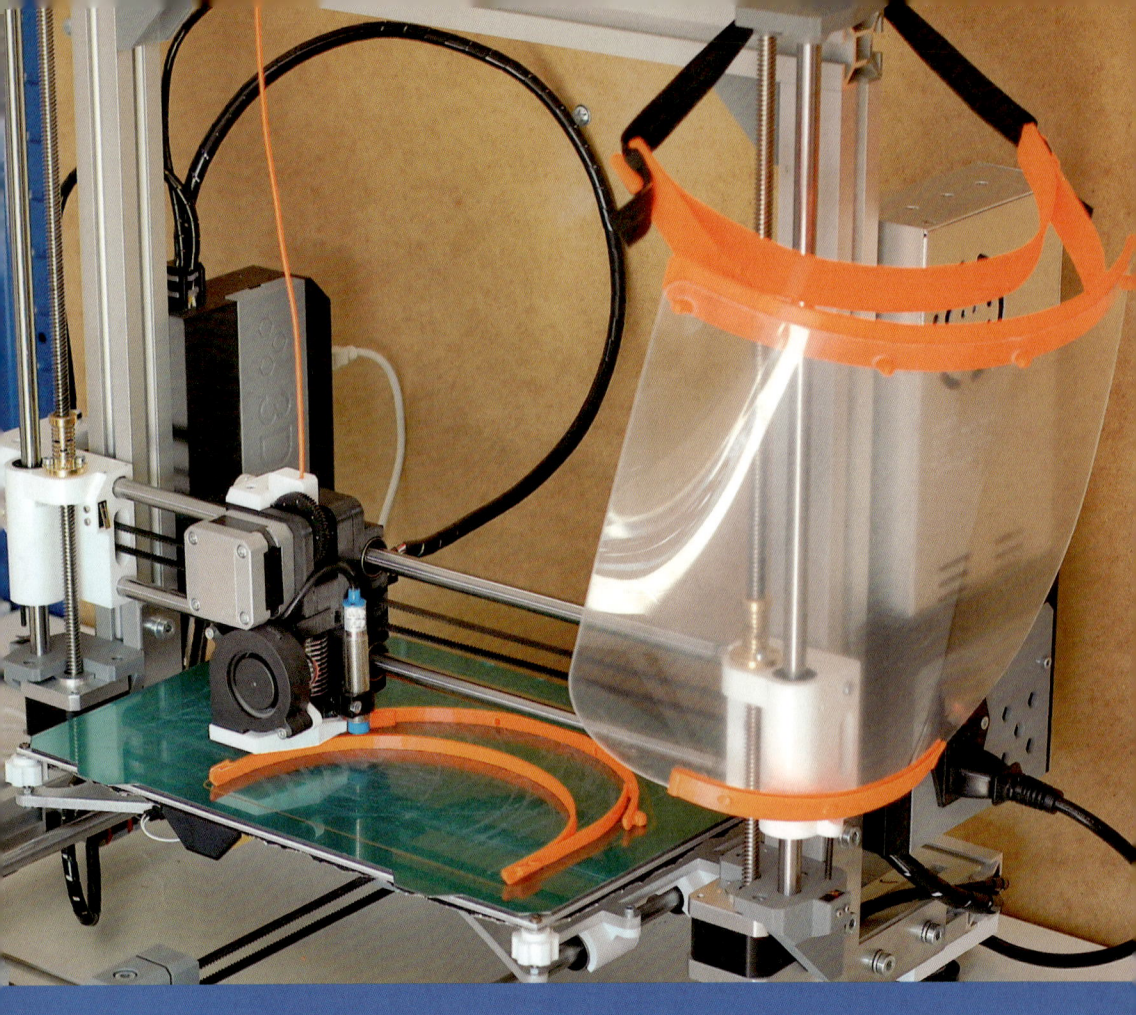

People with home 3D printers created parts for face shields during the COVID-19 pandemic.

face masks and face shields to block these droplets. But there were sometimes shortages of these products. People with 3D printers rose to the challenge.

They designed and printed new kinds of masks and shields. Companies also used 3D printing to make nasal swabs used to test for the disease.

An article in *Nature Reviews Materials* discussed the impact of 3D printing during the pandemic. The authors believed this technology was useful and important. They said, "In the heat of the COVID-19 pandemic, 3D printing has stepped up to become a vital technology to support improved health care and our general response to the emergency."[5]

CHAPTER FOUR

WHAT'S NEXT FOR 3D PRINTING IN HEALTH CARE?

Sometimes a patient's organs cannot be fixed. His heart, kidney, or liver may be failing. The patient needs an organ transplant. A surgeon takes a healthy organ from a donor. He puts it into the patient. These surgeries have come a long way.

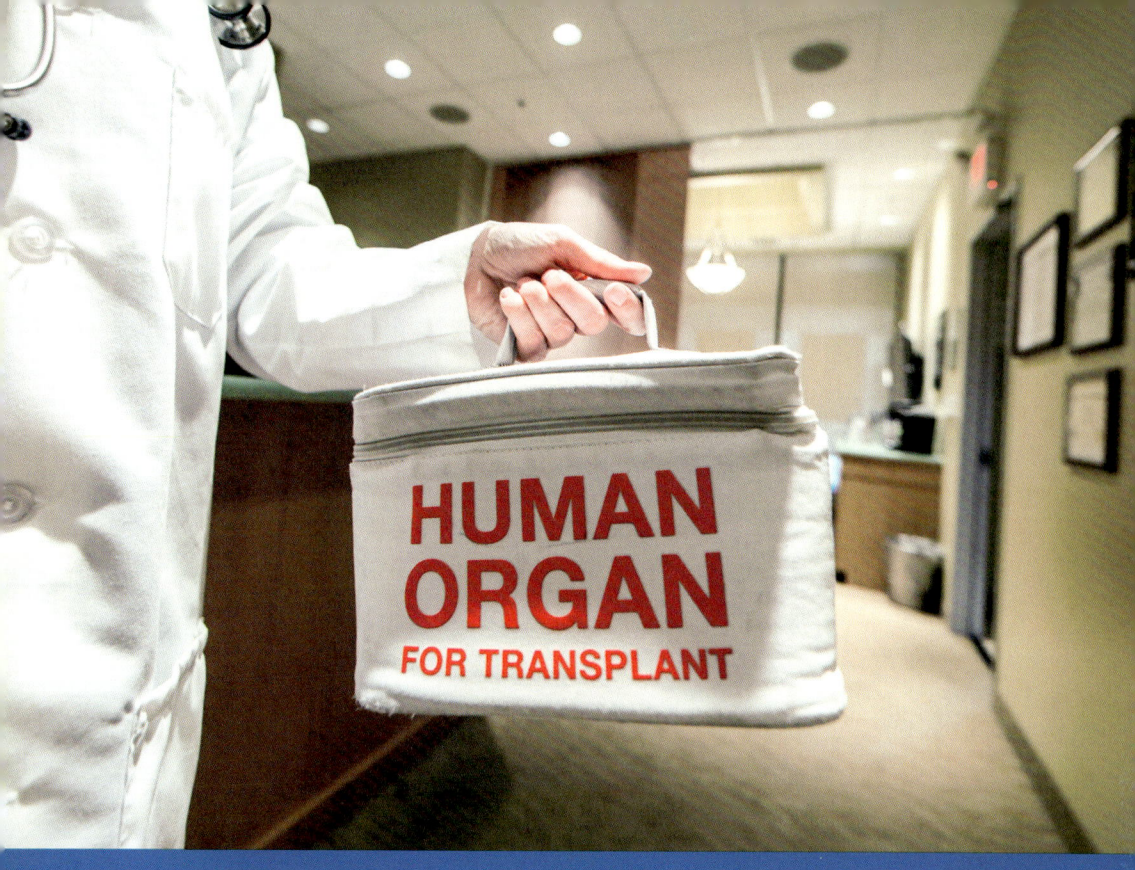

Transplanting organs involves transportation, rejection, and other challenges. Bioprinting could make things easier.

However, there are not enough donor organs for patients who need them. Donor organ tissue needs to match with the patient's tissue. Otherwise, the patient's body will reject the tissue. The donor organ will fail. Organ transplant patients must take medicine for the rest of their lives to prevent rejection.

Bioprinted organs could solve these problems. An organ could be printed when needed. The patient would not have to wait for a donor. The organ would be made from

TRANSPLANT WAITING LIST

In February 2021, more than 107,000 people in the United States were on donor organ waiting lists. But in the previous year, only about 39,000 people had received transplants. Many people were unable to get the organs they needed. Researchers hope that bioprinted organs will solve this problem in the future.

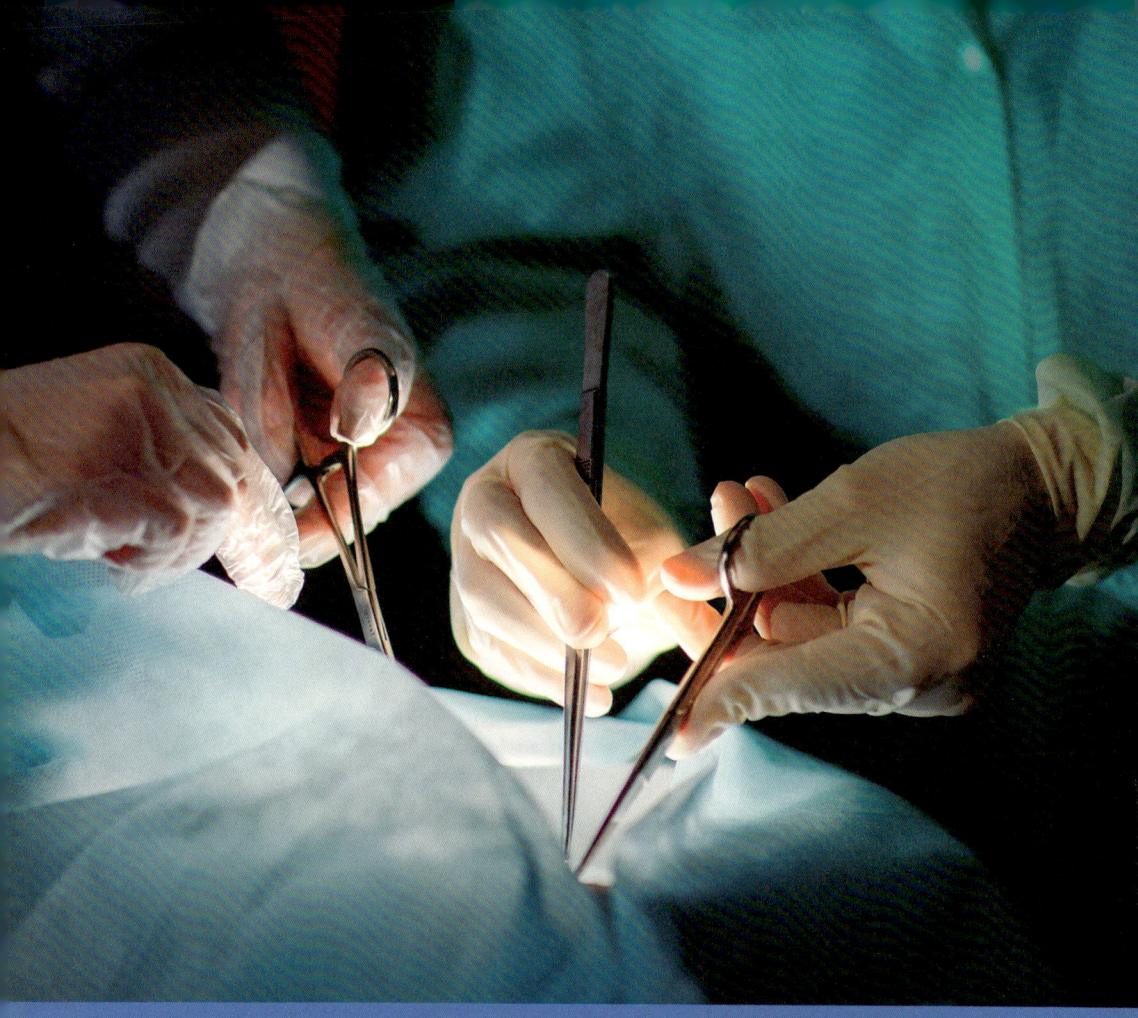

3D printed organs would change the world of organ transplants.

the patient's own cells. That means it would not be rejected. It could even be made to match the exact size and shape of the patient's old organ.

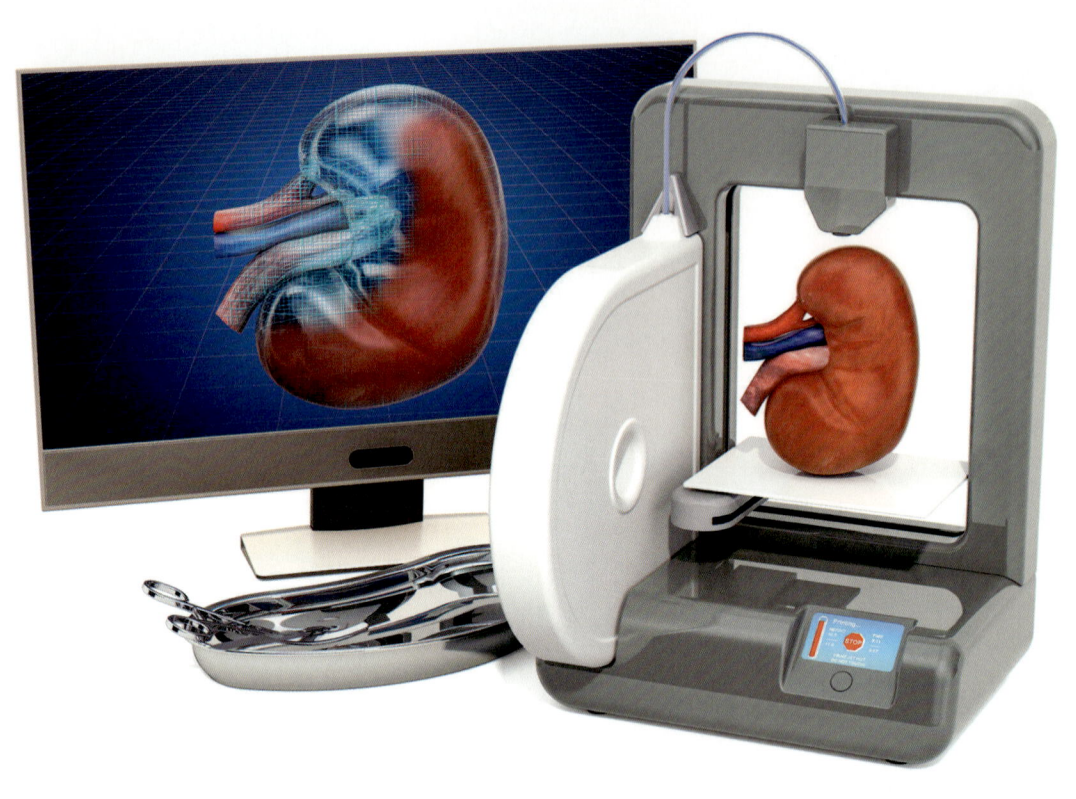

3D printing full organs is still in the future, but scientists are working toward this goal.

Making printed organ cells act like native cells is a challenge. Scientists are trying to bioprint with a patient's stem cells. Stem cells are able to grow into many different kinds of cells. After printing, the stem cells would grow into the needed type. Scientists have not yet bioprinted a heart, kidney, or liver that could be implanted. They continue to research how this could be done.

BLOOD VESSELS

There are about 100,000 miles (160,934 km) of blood vessels in the body. These vessels carry blood to organs. Printed organs must connect with them to work. Researchers are looking for ways to make **capillaries** to keep organs alive. They have already printed larger blood vessels. Making capillaries will bring scientists one step closer to replacement organs.

Dr. Monica Moya is a researcher in California. She uses bioprinting to make living blood vessels. Moya works to create small capillaries that grow on their own. Tubes of cells and other biomaterials are printed out around the blood vessels. Over time, capillaries develop. They connect with these tubes. This creates networks of blood vessels like those in the body.

Moya's goal is to use these vessels to keep an implanted organ alive. She explains, "We can put the cells in an environment where they know, 'I need to

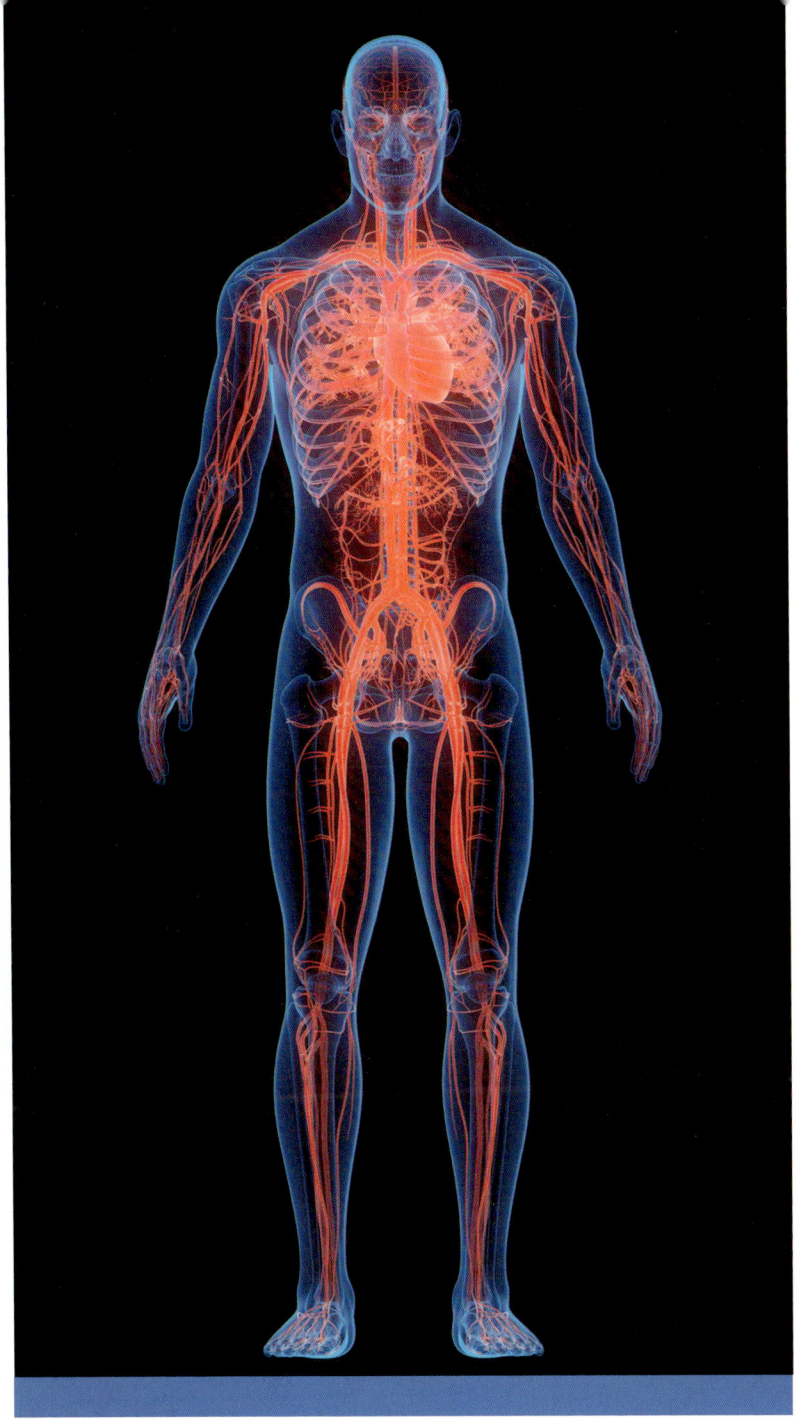

The body has an enormous network of blood vessels. Making implanted organs work with this system is a big challenge.

build blood vessels.' With this technology we guide . . . the biology."[6]

SKIN

Skin is the body's largest organ. Sometimes patients get bad burns on their skin. Doctors take healthy skin from another part of the body and graft it to the burn. In bad burn cases, the patient might not have enough healthy skin to graft. Researchers at WFIRM have developed a system to print skin grafts right onto burned skin. In a 2019 project, they demonstrated how this bioprinter could be used.

The system uses a scanner to map a patient's wound. It looks at the shape and depth of the wound. An inkjet printer then lays down the cells and other materials necessary to form human skin. Skin has many layers. The system places the right kinds of cells at the right depth.

ROBOTIC EXOSKELETON

Experts have developed a 3D printed prosthesis for children with muscle problems. The light, plastic device fits around the child's arms, torso, or legs. A set of resistance bands and metal bars provides strength. The device allows these children to stand, walk, and use their hands.

The goal is to build portable printers for use in field hospitals. Doctors would be able to print skin directly onto patients in need. This technology is still in the experimental stage. Researchers hope it will be widely available in the future.

HOPE FOR THE FUTURE

3D printing is already benefiting people in many ways. Doctors can make joint replacements, hearing aids, and braces that fit just right. Medical students and surgeons can use 3D printing to improve their skills. 3D printing even lets drugmakers test and manufacture medicines.

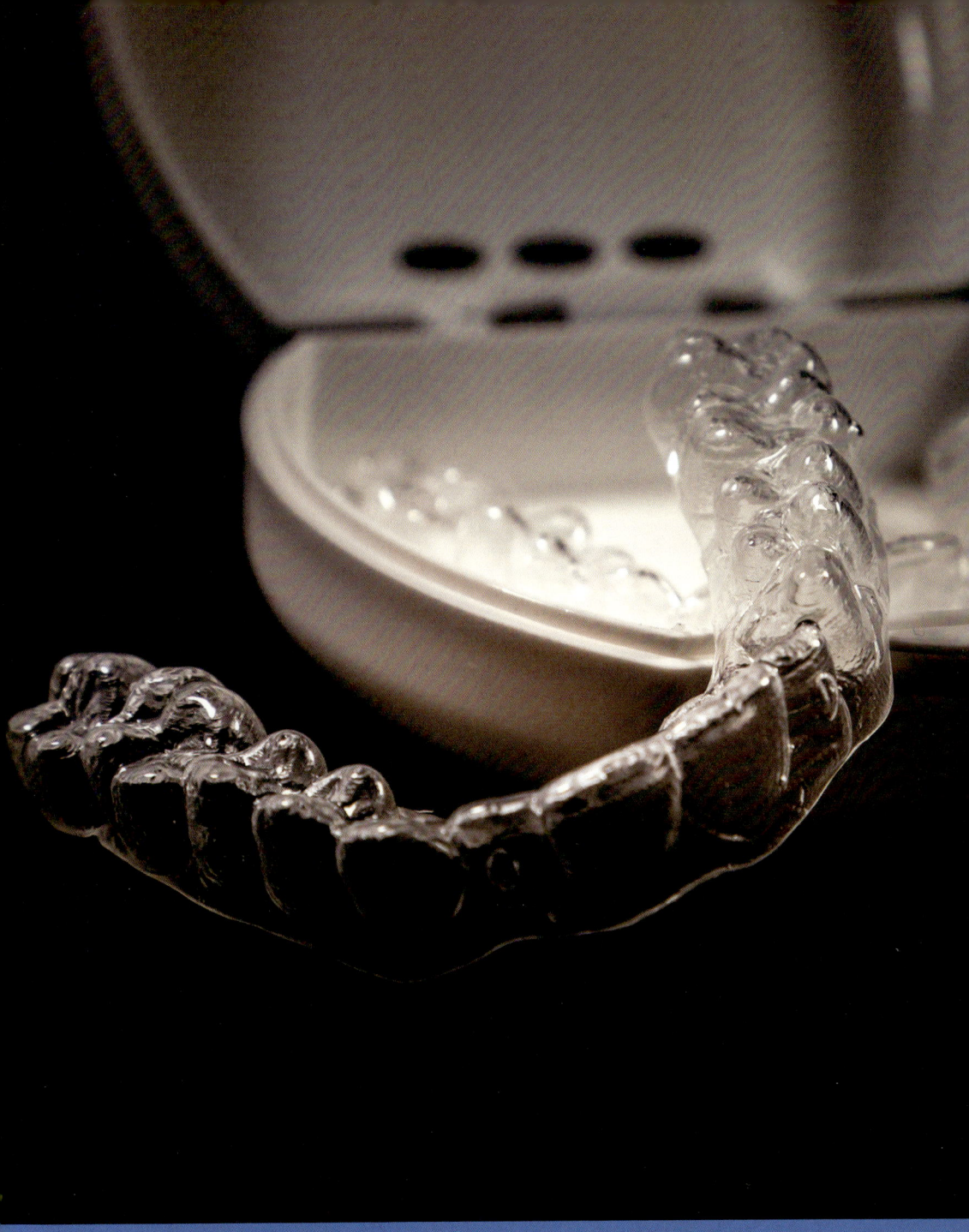

People around the world are using tooth-straightening devices created by 3D printers.

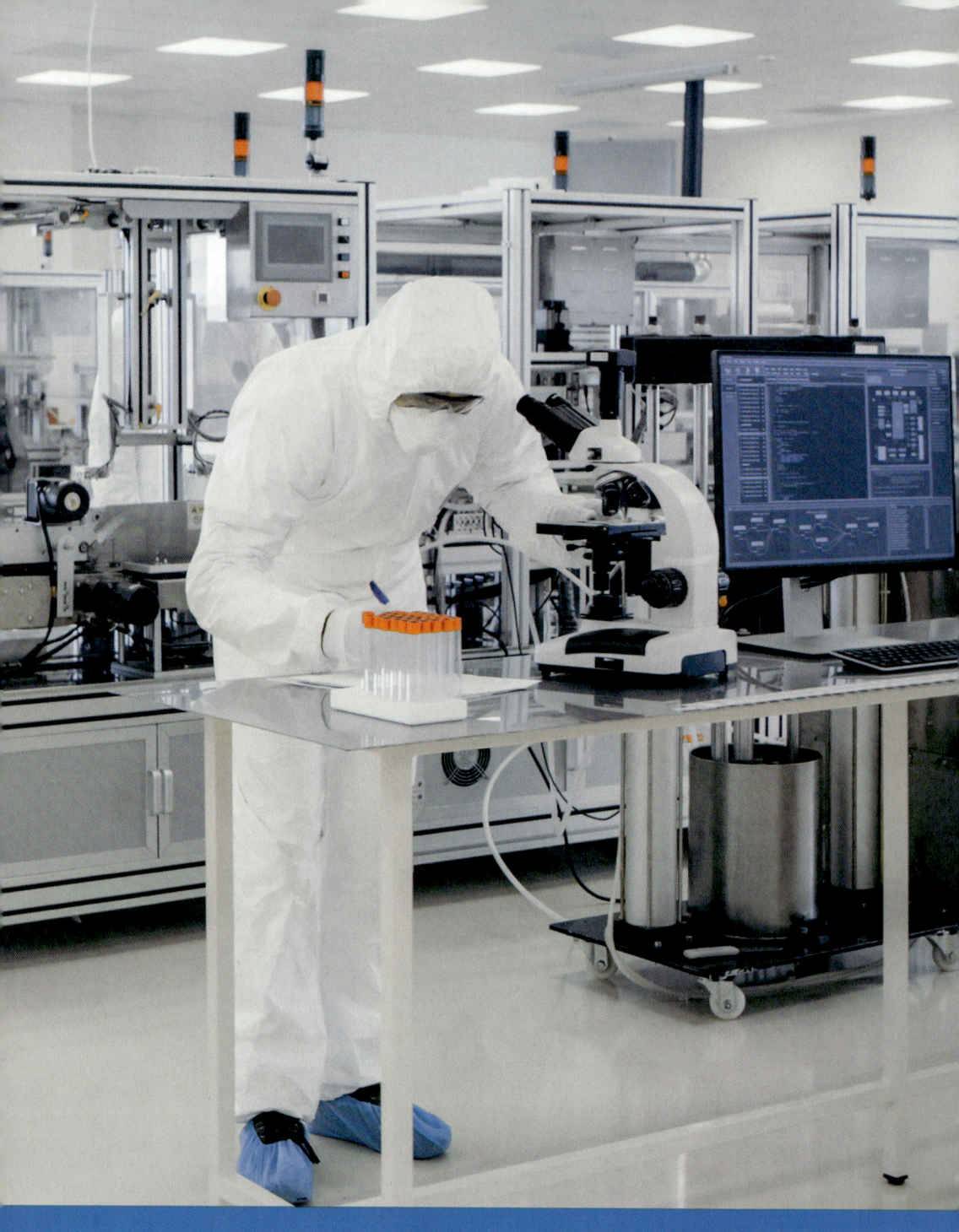

In medical labs around the world, researchers are making advances in 3D printing.

Scientists are hopeful that future advances will help even more people. They look forward to bioprinting working organs. Adam Feinberg works at Carnegie Mellon University. He says, "It is important to understand that there are many years of research yet to be done. But there should still be excitement that we're making real progress towards engineering functioning human tissues and organs."[7]

GLOSSARY

artificial
made by people

biomaterials
materials that can function alongside living cells and tissues

capillaries
the body's smallest type of blood vessels

cells
the smallest building blocks that make up living things

laser
a tightly focused beam of light

nutrients
the substances living things need to stay alive

porous
having small holes

reservoir
a container that holds a material

titanium
a very strong type of metal

SOURCE NOTES

CHAPTER ONE: WHAT IS THE HISTORY OF 3D PRINTING IN HEALTH CARE?

1. Quoted in Matthew Whitaker, "The History of 3D Printing in Healthcare," *The Bulletin*, June 12, 2015. https://publishing.rcseng.ac.uk.

2. Quoted in Vanesa Listek, "Dr. Anthony Atala Explains the Frontiers of Bioprinting for Regenerative Medicine at Wake Forest," *3D Print*, April 29, 2019. www.3dprint.com.

CHAPTER TWO: HOW DOES 3D PRINTING IN HEALTH CARE WORK?

3. Quoted in Sony Salzman, "3D-Printed Hearts with 'Beating' Tissue Could Ease Organ Donor Shortage," *NBC News*, September 23, 2019. www.nbcnews.com.

CHAPTER THREE: HOW ARE DOCTORS USING 3D PRINTING TODAY?

4. Quoted in "How 3D Printing and Modeling Are Changing Joint Replacement Surgery," *Yale Medicine*, July 26, 2019. www.yalemedicine.org.

5. Yi Ying Clarrisa Choong, et al., "The Global Rise of 3D Printing During the COVID-19 Pandemic," *Nature Reviews Materials*, August 12, 2020. www.nature.com.

CHAPTER FOUR: WHAT'S NEXT FOR 3D PRINTING IN HEALTH CARE?

6. Quoted in "Printing the Future: 3D Bioprinters and Their Uses," *Australian Academy of Science*, February 29, 2016. https://science.org.au.

7. Quoted in Anna MacDonald, "Bioprinting Organs—A Future Alternative to Organ Donation?" *Cell Science*, September 2, 2019. www.technologynetworks.com.

FOR FURTHER RESEARCH

BOOKS

Valerie Bodden, *3-D Printers*. Minneapolis, MN: Abdo Publishing, 2018.

Karen Latchana Kenney, *Cutting-Edge 3D Printing*. Minneapolis, MN: Lerner Publications, 2019.

Hal Marcovitz, *3-D Printing*. Chicago, IL: Norwood House Press, 2017.

INTERNET SOURCES

Eric Niiler, "Bio-printers Are Churning Out Living Fixes to Broken Spines," *Wired*, January 14, 2019. www.wired.com.

Ellen Rosen, "A Possible Weapon Against the Pandemic: Printing Human Tissue," *New York Times*, July 27, 2020. www.nytimes.com.

Matt Simon, "This Squishy 3D-Printed Human Heart Feels Like the Real Thing," *Wired*, November 23, 2020. www.wired.com.

WEBSITES

FDA: 3D Printing of Medical Devices
www.fda.gov/medical-devices/products-and-medical-procedures/3d-printing-medical-devices

The website of the US Food and Drug Administration has information about 3D printing of medical devices. It also features links to more resources about 3D printing.

Thingiverse
www.thingiverse.com/education

The Thingiverse website features 3D models that users can download and print at home or at the library.

3D Insider
https://3dinsider.com/3d-printing-for-kids/

This website features information about the history of 3D printing, how it works, and how people can start 3D printing their own objects.

INDEX

airways, 6–8
Atala, Anthony, 20–21, 42

bioink, 29, 31–33, 37–38
biomaterials, 13, 19, 20, 29, 66
bioprinters, 29–35, 38, 68
bladders, 20–21, 44
blood vessels, 25, 30, 35, 36, 65–68
Boland, Thomas, 22–24
bones, 30, 36, 44–49, 51, 52
braces, 51, 70

cartilage, 21, 26, 43, 44
casts, 51
computers, 7, 9, 15, 20, 23, 36
COVID-19, 56–59

drug manufacturing, 54–56
drug testing, 54

ears, 43–44
education, 18, 28, 52

Feinberg, Adam, 73

hearing aids, 51
hearts, 26, 44, 52, 60, 65
Hull, Charles, 14–16, 18

joints, 42, 44–47, 70

lasers, 15, 32–33, 47
Lewis, Jennifer, 39

medical scans, 7, 35–36, 43, 69
motors, 9, 33–34
Moya, Monica, 66–68

organs, 19–20, 30, 39, 40, 44, 52, 54, 60–65, 73

plastic, 10, 13, 14–16, 28, 30, 46, 51, 69
prosthetics, 25, 49–50, 69

skin, 21, 22, 44, 68–70

titanium, 46–47
training, 52–53

IMAGE CREDITS

Cover: © agefotostock/Alamy
5: © Aleksandr Ivasenko/
Shutterstock Images
7: © Sergey Ryzhov/
Shutterstock Images
9: © FabrikaSimf/Shutterstock Images
11: © asharkyu/Shutterstock Images
12: © stockddvideo/
Shutterstock Images
15: © sspopov/Shutterstock Images
17: © Joel Papalini/iStockphoto
21: © Lynn Hey/AP Images
23: © Wuttisak Promchoo/
Shutterstock Images
25: © asharkyu/Shutterstock Images
27: © The World in HDR/
Shutterstock Images
29: © Bas Nastassia/
Shutterstock Images
31: © Scharfsinn/Shutterstock Images
32: © Kirill Kallinikov/Sputnik/
AP Images
34: © Mikkel Juul Jensen/
Science Source
37: © Andrey_Popov/
Shutterstock Images
38: © Adrian Mars/
Shutterstock Images
41: © Bangkoker/Shutterstock Images
43: © Adrian Mars/
Shutterstock Images
46: © Monstar Studio/
Shutterstock Images
48: © Marina_Skoropadskaya/
Shutterstock Images
50: © Malikov Aleksandr/
Shutterstock Images
53: © SDI Productions/iStockphoto
55: © Cagkan Sayin/
Shutterstock Images
57: © Fotomay/Shutterstock Images
58: © Lucie Peclova/
Shutterstock Images
61: © photographereddie/iStockphoto
63: © David Tadevosian/
Shutterstock Images
64: © AlexLMX/iStockphoto
67: © magicmine/iStockphoto
71: © tigristiara/Shutterstock Images
72: © gorodenkoff/iStockphoto

ABOUT THE AUTHOR

Marne Ventura is the author of more than one hundred books for children. A former elementary school teacher, she holds a master's degree in Reading and Language Development from the University of California. Marne's nonfiction titles cover a wide range of topics, including STEM, arts and crafts, food and cooking, biographies, health, and survival. Her fiction series, the Worry Warriors, tells the story of four brave kids who learn to conquer their fears. Marne and her husband live on the central coast of California.